A Straight Talking Introduction to

Children's Mental
Health Problems

Sami Timimi

PCCS BOOKS
Ross-on-Wye

First published in 2009

PCCS BOOKS Ltd
2 Cropper Row
Alton Road
Ross-on-Wye
Herefordshire
HR9 5LA
UK
Tel +44 (0)1989 763900
www.pccs-books.co.uk

**A Straight Talking Introduction to
Children's Mental Health Problems**

A CIP catalogue record for this book is available from the British Library

ISBN 978 1 906254 15 5

Cover designed in the UK by Old Dog Graphics
Typeset in the UK by The Old Dog's Missus
Printed in the UK by Ashford Colour Press, Gosport, Hampshire

Contents

Introduction to the *Straight Talking* series

What are mental health problems?

Much of what is written and spoken about emotional distress or
mental health problems implies that they are illnesses. This can
lead us all too easily to believe that we no longer have to think
about mental health problems, because illness is best left to
doctors. They are the illness experts, and psychiatrists are the
doctors who specialise in mental illness. This series of books is
different because we don't think that all mental health problems
should be automatically regarded as illnesses.

If mental health problems aren't necessarily illnesses, it means
that the burden of responsibility for distress in our lives should not
be entirely shouldered by doctors and psychiatrists. All citizens
have a responsibility, however small, in creating a world where
everyone has a decent opportunity to live a fulfilling life. This is a
contentious idea, but one which we want to advance alongside the
dominant medical view.

Rather than accept that solutions to mental health problems
are 'owned' by the medical profession, we will take a good look at
alternatives which involve the users of psychiatric services, their
carers, families, friends and other 'ordinary people' taking control
of their own lives. One of the tools required in order to become
active in mental health issues, whether your own or other people's,
is knowledge. This series of books is a starting point for anyone
who wants to know more about mental health.

How these books are written

We want these books to be understandable, so we use everyday
language wherever possible. The books could have been almost
completely jargon-free, but we thought that including some
technical and medical terms would be helpful. Most doctors,

psychiatrists and psychologists use the medical model of mental illness and manuals to help them diagnose mental health problems. The medical model and the diagnostic manuals use a particular set of terms to describe what doctors think of as 'conditions'. Although these words aren't very good at describing individual people's experiences, they are used a lot in psychiatric and psychological services, so we thought it would be helpful to define these terms as we went along and use them in a way that might help readers understand what the professionals mean. We don't expect that psychiatrists and psychologists and others working in mental health services will stop using medical terminology (although we think it might be respectful for them to drop it when talking to their patients and their families), so these books should help you get used to, and learn *their* language.

At the end of the book there are endnotes; these will not be important to everyone, but they do tell the reader where information – a claim about effectiveness, an argument for or against, or a quotation – has come from so you can follow it up if you wish.

Being realistic and reassuring

Our aim is to be realistic – neither overly optimistic nor pessimistic. Things are nearly always more complicated than we would like them to be. Honest evaluations of mental health problems, of what might cause them, of what can help, and of what the likely outcome might be, are, like so much in life, somewhere in between. For the vast majority of people it would be wrong to say that they have an illness from which they will never recover. But it would be equally wrong to say that they will be completely unchanged by the distressing thoughts and feelings they are having. Life is an accumulation of experiences. There is usually no pill, or any other treatment for that matter, that will take us back to 'how we were before'. There are many things we can do (and we will be looking at lots of them in this series) in collaboration with doctors, psychiatrists, psychologists, counsellors, indeed everyone working in mental health services, with the help of our friends and family, or on our own, which stand a good chance of helping us feel better and build a constructive life with hope for the future.

Of course, we understand that the experiences dealt with in these books can sometimes be so overwhelming, confusing and terrifying that people will try to escape from them by withdrawing, going mad or even by trying to kill themselves. This happens when our usual coping strategies fail us. We accept that killing oneself is, in some circumstances, a rational act – that for the person in question it can make a lot of sense. Nonetheless, we believe that much of the distress that underpins such an extreme course of action, from which there can be no turning back, is avoidable. For this reason, all of the books in this series point towards realistic hope and recovery.

Debates

There is no single convenient answer to many of the most important questions explored in these books. No matter how badly we might wish for a simple answer, what we have is a series of debates, or arguments more like, between stakeholders and there are many stakeholders whose voices demand space in these books. We use the word 'stakeholders' here because service users, carers, friends, family, doctors, psychologists, psychiatrists, nurses and other workers, scientists in drug companies, therapists, indeed all citizens, have a stake in how our society understands and deals with problems of mental health. It is simultaneously big business and intimately personal, and many things in between. As we go along, we try to explain how someone's stake in distress (including our own, where we can see it), whether business or personal, can influence their experience and judgement.

Whilst we want to present competing (sometimes opposing) viewpoints, we don't want to leave the reader high and dry to evaluate complicated debates on their own. We will try to present reasonable conclusions which might point in certain directions for personal action. Above all, though, we believe that knowledge is power and that the better informed you are, even though the information might be conflicting, the more able you will be to make sound decisions.

It's also useful to be reminded that the professionals involved in helping distressed people are themselves caught in the same flow of conflicting information. It is their *job*, however, to interpret it in our service, so that the best solutions are available to as many people as possible. You may have noticed that the word 'best' brings with it certain challenges, not least of all, what we mean when we use this term. Perhaps the best means the most effective? However, even using words like 'effective' doesn't completely clear up the puzzle. An effective treatment could be the one which returns someone to work quickly, if you are an employer, or one which makes someone feel happier and more calm, if they are your son or daughter. Readers will also know from recent press coverage that the National Institute for Health and Clinical Excellence (NICE) which evaluates and recommends treatments, keeps one eye on the budget, so 'effective' might mean 'cost effective' to some people. This brings us to evidence.

Evidence

Throughout these books there will be material which we will present as 'evidence'. This is one of the most contentious terms to be found in this series. One person's evidence is another person's fanciful mythology and yet another person's oppressive propaganda. Nevertheless the term crops up increasingly in everyday settings, most relevantly when we hear of 'evidence-based practice'. The idea behind this term is that the treatments psychologists and psychiatrists offer should be those that work. Crudely put, there should be some evidence that, say, talking about problems, or taking a prescribed drug, actually helps people to feel better. We encounter a real problem however, when trying to evaluate this evidence, as the books will demonstrate. We will try not to discount any 'evidence' out of hand, but we will evaluate it, and we will do this with a bias towards scientific evaluation.

The types of evidence that will be covered in these books, along with their positive and negative points, include the following.

Research methods, numbers and statistics

On the one hand, the logic of most research is simple, but on the other hand, the way things have to be arranged to avoid bias in the results can lead to a perplexing system of measurements. Even the experts lose the sense of it sometimes. We'll try to explain the logic of studies, but almost certainly leave out the details. You can look these up yourself if you wish.

The books in this series look at research into a wide range of issues regarding mental health problems, including the experience of distress, what is known about the causes of problems, and their prevention and treatment. Different research methods are more or less appropriate for each of these areas, so we will be looking at different types of research as we go along. We say this now because many readers may be most familiar with studies into the *effective treatments* of distress, and we want to emphasise that there are many credible and valid sources of essential information about distress that are sometimes overlooked.

You may have come across the idea that some research methods are 'better' than others – that they constitute a 'gold standard'. In the case of research into the effectiveness of different treatments, the gold standard is usually considered to be 'randomised controlled trials' (RCTs). In simple terms, RCTs are complex (and often very expensive) experiments in which a group of individuals who all suffer from the same problem are randomly allocated to a treatment or a 'control' condition (at its simplest, no treatment at all) to see whether the treatment works. We are not necessarily convinced that RCTs always *are* the best way of conducting research into effective treatments, but they are, at the present time, the method given most credence by bodies which control funding, such as the National Health Service's National Institute of Health and Clinical Excellence (NICE), so we need to understand them.

Personal experience

Personal experience is an important source of evidence to the extent that nowadays, people who have suffered debilitating psychiatric distress are sometimes called 'experts by experience'.

Personal stories provide an essential counterbalance to the impersonal numbers and statistics often found in research projects such as RCTs. Whilst not everyone is average, by definition, most people are. Balancing the average results obtained from RCTs with some personal stories helps complete the picture and is now widely accepted to the extent that it has given birth to the new field of 'survivor research'.

Understanding contexts

Widening our view to include the families and lives of people, and the cultural, economic, social and political settings in which we live completes the picture. Mental health problems are connected to the conditions in which we all live, just as much as they are connected to our biology. From the start we want readers to know that, if there is one message or model which the books are trying to get across, it is that problems in mental health are more often than not the result of complex events in the environments in which we live and our reactions to them. These reactions can also be influenced by our biology or the way we have learned to think and feel. Hopefully these books will help disentangle the puzzle of distress and provide positive suggestions and hope for us all, whether we work in the system, currently have mental health problems ourselves, are caring for someone or are friends with someone who has.

We hope that readers of these books will feel empowered by what they learn, and thereby more able to get the best out of mental health services. It would be wonderful if our efforts, directly or indirectly, influence the development of services that effectively address the emotional, social and practical needs of people with mental health problems.

Richard Bentall
Pete Sanders
April 2009

Chapter 1
The work of culture

Eleven-year-old Afia has found it difficult to settle into her new secondary school, is crying before she goes to school and has started to develop habits like washing her hands for long periods and asking her parents to disinfect objects around the house.

Eight-year-old Kyle's parents are regularly called in to see his teachers because of his disruptive behaviour in class.

Fourteen-year-old Hannah has always been a conscientious but shy pupil. She has been slowly reducing the amount she eats and hasn't had a period for five months now.

Fifteen-year-old Jason has become increasingly withdrawn, refuses to go to school, complains of 'voices in his head' and spends most of his time playing an online computer game.

Ten-year-old Tariq gets easily upset and fights a lot with his sister. He sometimes cries about missing his father who left the family home a year ago.

Five-year-old Zara has become clingy to her mother and is so scared of dogs that she refuses to walk anywhere.

Many things cause us to feel mental distress, and distress presents in many different ways. If there was an easy, foolproof, scientifically supported, simple way of approaching these diverse presentations, I would be delighted to get straight down to that task right now. Indeed according to many psychiatric textbooks I could do this and start talking about how we categorise, assess and then treat these mental problems. However, I believe this would leave you, the reader, with a seriously incomplete picture of the difficulty involved in such a simple approach – attractive and reassuring as such an approach may appear. Therefore I am first going to have to ask you to be a little patient, as before we get to the the heart of the matter, I am first going to explain why I don't believe it is helpful to jump straight to the 'assessment, diagnosis, treatment' approach.

It can feel confusing and bewildering, not to mention frustrating, for any parent trying to make sense of their child's problems and how to help them. It is likely that a parent or young person struggling with distress or difficult behaviours that cause distress can encounter a variety of often contradictory messages about what's going on and what to do about it. You might read something in an article in a magazine that gets you wondering if the problems are caused by an illness like Attention Deficit Hyperactivity Disorder (ADHD), autism, or childhood depression. You may see a TV programme that gets you worried that their diet is wrong or that too much time playing computer games is affecting the mind of your troubled youngster. You may worry that it's your parenting or family breakdown that is the problem, and feel guilty and ashamed every time the school calls you in to discuss the latest episode of 'bad' behaviour. How do you make sense of your own particular individual distress? How do you sift through all these different ideas to find the one that will be most useful to you and your family?

Facing these questions means that we have to consider what sense we make of the evidence that is presented to us and the confusing variety of opinions from both professionals and non-professionals that we have to deal with. It is the different meanings we give to the facts that we have which have caused many of the controversies and confusion that exist with regard to the various forms of childhood distress that attract the various labels (such as ADHD, autism and childhood depression).

To help guide you on this 'making sense of childhood distress' journey, my starting point is thus not the science (which I will come to later) but the issue of how we make sense of the science. This means that we first have to depart from the language of pure science and objective facts into the territory of the humanities (which includes areas such as philosophy, cultural studies, anthropology, sociology and many aspects of psychology). A humanities perspective will help us to try and understand some of the human, social, cultural and political processes that are involved when we come to make sense of the world around us. This means looking at complexity from a 'subjective' rather than a purely 'objective' point of view.

Let me give you a simple example from everyday life. I recently picked up a lovely ripe pomegranate in the supermarket. My nine-year-old daughter was later persuaded to try a bit when I was eating it. Now there are many objective things I could say about this pomegranate. For example, I could weigh it, measure its volume, the thickness of its skin, the chemical constituents held within it, the types of sugars, vitamins and minerals and relative amounts of each and so on. I could carry out a scientific study of the life cycle of a pomegranate from seed to tree to flowering to pollination to the growth of the fruit and so on. All of this is of course useful information, enlarging my understanding of the natural world as well as informing me about how healthy (or otherwise) it is for me and my children to eat this fruit.

How far, however, can this objective, scientific approach capture the different experience that my daughter and I had when we then ate this pomegranate? For my daughter the pomegranate was not a fruit she was familiar with and so she approached it tentatively, perhaps already imagining that she was not going to like it. My daughter tried a couple of pieces from the pomegranate and indeed decided she did not like the texture or the taste. For me the pomegranate had an altogether different significance that weaves into the different personal history that I carry. Pomegranate was a favourite fruit of mine when I was growing up in Iraq. When pomegranates were in season I would eat copious amounts. Sometimes just the very act of peeling away the thin, rubbery lining that divides the seeds in the fruit into compartments brings back memories of my childhood, long summer days during the school holidays spent with one of my cousins who also loved the pomegranate. We both used to like picking out the seeds, putting them in a bowl and sprinkling a bit of sugar on them. Just remembering this brings a smile to my face.

So if we simply stick with studying the objective qualities of the pomegranate (like its weight, nutritional content etc.) we will miss a huge and important part of, arguably, the very thing that makes us human, our subjective experience of it. It is that unique context of our personal history and how this interacts with our wider social and cultural contexts, which structures our sense of meaning, values and what it is we consider important to us throughout our lives. Just as the pomegranate has a particular meaning for me, which often makes me buy a pomegranate when I see one in a shop, so it is likely that for my daughter pomegranates will have a very different meaning in her life – one which will probably make her behave rather differently to me when she sees a pomegranate amongst the fruits at the grocers. This is not to say that objective knowledge about the pomegranate becomes redundant or loses its usefulness or relevance when it comes to deciding whether to eat a pomegranate or not. However, it is to say that only by incorporating sensitivity to understanding the subjective that we can hope to begin to make sense of human behaviour, emotions and experience.

One of the problems with the type of thinking that promotes the idea that some children suffer from medical conditions such as ADHD or childhood depression is that it comes from a particular, philosophical approach to science that does exactly what I have described above – it attempts to find only 'objective' knowledge and marginalises the importance of understanding the subjective.

Our broader political, cultural and economic context interacts with our personal history to create our subjective beliefs and values, which in turn shape how we behave and perceive the world. Our beliefs and values in turn influence the practice of science, affecting what we choose to investigate and how we then interpret the results of what we have investigated. This continuous interaction we sometimes refer to as a 'dynamic'. When we talk about the dynamics of a situation we are referring to interacting processes that form certain patterns.

Culture and social construction

This is where the concept of culture is useful even though different people mean different things when they use the word 'culture'. Here is one definition of culture that I have found useful: 'The peculiar and distinctive way of life of a group, the meanings, values and ideas embodied in institutions, in social relations, in systems of belief, in customs, in the uses of objects and material life … the "maps of meaning" that make things intelligible to its members.'[1] In other words: a set of beliefs and a 'way of doing things' that a certain group of people have in common.

This means that we can examine and talk about 'culture' at many different levels as we can draw an imaginary boundary around groups of people that have something in common in many different ways; from small groups right up to sets of nations and whole regions. So, for example, we can talk about the culture of a particular family, a particular profession, a particular city, a particular country, a particular religion, a particular continent even. Each of these groupings will contain 'something' in common to mark them out from other similar groupings (like a different family, a different profession, a different religion and so on). This of course also means we have to be very careful when we talk about 'the culture' of a particular group, as each group is made up of individuals who are going to possess significant differences between them and will simultaneously belong to several different possible cultural groupings (for example, if we were to take a city as our starting cultural grouping, people within this city will also belong to different families, professional groups, religions, speak different languages and so on). This means we always must be careful not to 'tar everyone with the same brush'; not to stereotype.

The process by which different cultures develop a set of beliefs and values that guide the way they subsequently behave in the world and in relation to each other is often summarised by the term 'social construction'. In other words, groups of people who share a common cultural set of values and beliefs are said to socially construct their understanding of the world around them.

Let me give you a simple example in relation to a child who is perceived to be displaying persistent poor behaviour. As a generalisation (remembering my warning about stereotyping) we can see that different cultures will interpret the reasons for this differently and so go about the task of trying to modify this differently. In the West today, it may lead to a concern that the child has a medical condition and so a visit to the doctor may be organised that may eventually result in a diagnosis of ADHD or something similar and possibly the prescription of medication. In many other parts of the world and amongst some religious groups, because they have a different set of beliefs about children and about how the world works, a concern might be that the child is possessed by some supernatural entity. This belief will lead to a different strategy, for example a traditional healer or religious leader may be consulted and certain rituals may then be prescribed. I am not making any value judgement about which of the above two is 'better', just illustrating that if we 'socially construct' our world differently then how we understand a problem and what we do about it will also be different.

Of course social construction is nothing more than a useful idea and real life is much more complicated than can be summarised with a single term. A person's view of the world is going to be influenced by many things, not just the beliefs and values that they have absorbed from whatever cultural groups they have been a part of. Thus, individuals' perception of the world is likely to be shaped by a complex and continuing interaction between their biology (for example, inherited personality traits), their own personal history (for example, trauma and abuse during childhood is thought to have many long-term consequences on the way a person then perceives and behaves in relationships during the rest of their lives), as well as the different cultural groups whose values and beliefs a person has absorbed.

Meaning and values

Before going on to discuss the different cultural 'stories' (or social constructs) that exist about childhood distress, I would like to pause briefly and consider further the importance of how we interpret the meaning and significance of whatever version of the story we choose. This is because different meanings lead you to act in different ways.

Let me give you an example of a common presentation from a typical child psychiatric outpatient clinic:

> James is a seven-year-old boy who is described by his parents as 'very active'. When he was four years old, a nursery teacher reported that he was very active and had limited play with other children. His teacher at school now reports that he is not keeping up with either reading or mathematics and that he fidgets a lot. His parents report that he is easily bored and so tends to flit from one activity to another, but when given the chance spends a lot of time playing a computer game that he likes.

If I, as a doctor, decide that this young person is experiencing problems because he is suffering from a disorder of his brain called 'ADHD' then it may well result in me deciding to prescribe medication for this young person. If, on the other hand, I interpret his problems as being due to nutritional imbalances then I might prescribe supplements instead. However, I may choose to interpret James's behaviour as being within the normal spectrum that I expect for children of his age, in which case this might lead me to work with his parents and teachers to try and influence their perception of him and so reduce the amount of worry or concern they have. As all three may be perfectly plausible alternatives, which route I choose to go down says a lot about me as a practitioner and the value system I have that guides my choices and influences my interpretation of the evidence.

To help understand the potential consequences of the value judgements we make, let me cite one area of dispute around the most common child psychiatric disorder diagnosis – that of ADHD. In this particular argument (most noted in an ongoing dispute with a series of articles criticising each other, between two heavyweights in the field – Russell Barkley and Thom Hartmann)[2] both sides accept the idea that ADHD-type behaviours are primarily the result of biological processes. However one side (the Russell Barkley camp) sees this biological process as something that causes an undesirable deficit and disability and thus believes that these behaviours should be viewed as a medical disease, called ADHD, and which thus needs medical treatment. The other side (the Thom Hartmann camp) views ADHD-type behaviours as being down to a 'difference' in biological make-up that can also bring several advantages and desirable qualities to the individual and thus it should not be classified as a medical disease.

So what are the potential implications of these two views? Let's look at the arguments from the Thom Hartmann camp (to which my views are more closely aligned, hence my analysis is necessarily going to be biased in favour of this view). What this camp point out is that studies on children believed to have ADHD are more interested in areas where these children perform poorly compared to non-ADHD children and that they rarely look at those areas of ability where 'ADHD' children may actually outperform non-ADHD children such as, for example, in their ability to outscore their peers in one of the new, high-stimulation video games or on a skateboard. In other words the idea that ADHD is a medical disease shapes how the research is then conducted in such a way that it is already 'primed' to discover that ADHD children are 'losers'.[3]

This then takes us to a related question of whether there is any evidence to suggest that viewing ADHD-type behaviours as being the product of a biological difference that is sometimes advantageous to that individual is available. One answer comes in the peculiar form of claims that are made that many famous and successful people had (or have) ADHD. I say peculiar as this can be interpreted as evidence that they were (or are) living proof that their biology was not (or is not) causing a disabling disease state in their brain, as it is their mental talents that have caused them to excel.[4]

One implication of this line of thinking is that if we were to provide education that acknowledges the differences in the way people learn, we might soon be tapping a source of creativity that could be useful to our entire society. At the individual level it could help us think more positively about the attributes and strengths of young people with problems that can be called ADHD, rather than start on the path of focusing on their inadequacies. It would also require that we open ourselves up to the possibility that the kinds of skills we reward (particularly in schools) today may not be the only worthwhile skills. At the collective level this can lead us to ask some taxing political questions about whether the way we organise our society and education system is part of the problem that must first change.

When such questions are on the agenda, the rapid rise in our labelling of children as having a disability called 'ADHD' begins to look more like a symptom of a 'dysfunctional' society, than a growing realisation about a previously unrecognised disease.

For those who believe that ADHD is a medical disease that is genetically inherited (the Barkley camp), the implication is that such individuals are genetically dysfunctional and less evolved than the rest of us, and thus they are placed in a position of dependence upon experts tasked with researching their 'problems' and developing 'treatments' for these. In a caring society, the experts who then do the 'diagnosing' and 'treating' become the group endowed with the positive attributes of health, knowledge, intelligence and kindness, for it is these professionals whom we then need to rely on to come and 'save' these children from themselves, and who can also bring peace and happiness to families and schools. Of course many parents, teachers and indeed young people report great benefits from such an approach, with the young person getting extra services, and the label having appeared to provide an explanatory framework for their problems. However, the person diagnosed with ADHD is now seen as having a disability that limits their capacity to make a positive contribution to culture and society – particularly if they are not 'treated' so that they can get 'rid' of their ADHD.

But what if society wasn't caring? What are the implications then? Would there be a call for adults diagnosed with ADHD not to have children, for fear that this 'defect' will continue to spread? Even if society claims to be caring, does this extend to all sections of the population? Does the reality of living in a culture based around economic need for profit, which places money before people, mean that despite our claims of being caring, we are (as a culture) intolerant of children who will be a financial burden? Does this mean that the social control of children has become more important to our culture than nurturing and caring for them?

These are more than just interesting academic questions. As I detailed in one of my books[5] it was a mixture of poor science implying genetic dysfunction and the tendency to try and deal with social problems by the apparently 'scientific' approach of medicine that led to the emergence of the philosophy of eugenics and attempts to eradicate these perceived 'bad genes' from society. This led to hundreds of thousands in North America and Europe being forcibly sterilised and eventually to tens of thousands of 'mental' patients being killed in gas chambers in Nazi Germany, all under the active and willing supervision of doctors who perceived themselves as conducting important 'treatments' for the good of society.

Cultures across time and across the globe

Hopefully you are beginning to appreciate that the way we 'socially construct' emotional and behavioural problems has an enormous impact on what we then choose to do and on how the child (and those caring for her/him) views her/himself. This in turn can have an enormous impact on many aspects of that child's future and indeed on society as a whole. Having made this point I hope you are beginning to understand that if emotional and behavioural problems are socially constructed, then so must our beliefs about what should be considered 'normal' in a child. After all our ideas of what is 'abnormal' are shaped by our ideas about what is 'normal'. So the next stage in building up my arguments about the importance of having a cultural understanding is to examine the many different ideas that exist or have existed about childhood and the task of child rearing.

If we look back at the history of childhood in Western culture we find that each historical period creates its own ideas about what normal childhood and child-rearing methods should be like. Each historical period's ideas about childhood are not simply abandoned but we find that fragments from each period are included in the next period's ideas of childhood. Looking at the history of childhood in any culture (as well as between cultures) we can see that our ideas about what makes a normal or abnormal child and/or child-rearing practices are thus neither timeless nor universal, but instead rooted in the past and reshaped in the present.

In 1962 the historian Philippe Aries published a book called *Centuries of Childhood*.[6] It had a major impact in academic circles, particularly because of the boldness of its basic conclusion – that in medieval society childhood simply did not exist. An earlier author, Norbert Elias, had already anticipated Aries's arguments in his 1939 book *The Civilizing Process*,[7] in which Elias argues that the visible difference between children and adults (psychologically and socially) increases in the course of the (as Elias saw it) 'civilising' process – in other words the more 'civilised' we become the more we treat children differently and give children different roles to adults (remember he was writing at a time before globalisation where the European rulers were viewed as more 'civilised' than the citizens of their Empires). However, Aries's interpretation of the evidence was much more radical.

Aries argued that the modern idea of childhood as a separate life stage emerged in Europe between the fifteenth and eighteenth centuries, at the same time as modern ideas of family, home, privacy and individuality were developing. He suggested that before the fifteenth century in Europe children past the dependent age of infancy were seen simply as miniature adults, implying that they had the same expectations and social roles as adults (for example being expected to work and not having any separate social institutions solely for children such as school). Aries was not saying that this is necessarily a bad thing; if anything he was suggesting the reverse, that modern Western culture insists on a period of 'quarantine' through educational and other similar institutions, before allowing young people to join society. Even if we modify Aries's bold idea and acknowledge that every known society has its own beliefs and practices that in some respect mark off children from adults, the importance of his book is the understanding that what we consider to be 'normal' childhood is largely socially constructed and these constructions of childhood tend to be socially and historically specific.

When we look at the history of childhood in the West we can see changes occurring in all aspects of childhood and child rearing, further supporting the contention that childhood and child rearing are primarily socially constructed. For example, in medieval Europe, child rearing was seen as being a mother's responsibility for the first seven or so years of that child's life. However, during the Renaissance period in fifteenth century Italy, the emphasis began to change and the father–child relationship was now seen as the most important in child rearing. It was the father's responsibility to choose and hire a wet nurse, to watch over their children's development and to thoughtfully interpret their child's actions so as to understand and shape their future. An influential writer at this time was Dutchman Desiderius Erasmus. Erasmus placed considerable emphasis on early education and attacked those who, in his view, allowed children to be pampered by their mothers or wet nurses out of what he saw as a false spirit of tenderness. Instead he thought fathers had to take control of their children's (in particular their sons') upbringing, in order to develop their child's character in a way that would, in his view, bring them closer to reflecting the 'divine'.[8]

Then in the eighteenth century, the followers of Jean Jacques Rousseau attacked the traditions of the time that encouraged fathers to take charge of child rearing, insisting that fathers' ambition and harshness were more harmful to a child than the 'blind' affection of mothers. Rousseau asserted that children have a right to be happy in childhood and even went on to suggest that childhood may be the best time of life. With this Rousseau inspired the 'romantic movement' gaining a foothold in popular culture by the end of the eighteenth century, mothers regained the predominance they held in the Middle Ages and child rearing once again became a predominantly female occupation.[9]

So, in the example above, we can see that in the space of a few hundred years, the dominant belief about who should be the most important parent around whom the task of child rearing should revolve changed from mothers to fathers and then back to mothers again. There are many similar examples of beliefs about children and child rearing switching from one pole to the other. As well as visions of normal and abnormal childhood changing within cultures over time, many differences can be seen between different cultures and the varying traditions throughout the world.

As mentioned earlier it is a mistake to assume that understanding cultural 'trends' and traditions are sufficient to understand the individual from any particular group. That is the path to stereotyping. However, it is also a grave mistake (and one in my experience more likely to happen) to assume that there is one universal standard for measuring what is a normal (and therefore abnormal) childhood and one universal standard for how to parent. If we are to help all parents make sense of what might be a helpful way to view a difficult or distressed child, I can think of many worse places to start than appreciating this point. It is very common to feel guilty about what we do as parents, just as it has become very common to worry about our children's development. Knowing how difficult it is to pinpoint the 'normal' or 'right' way to do child rearing can at least reassure us that there is 'more than one way to skin a cat' as the rather gruesome saying goes.

For example in many non-Western cultures you are likely to encounter more immediate gratification of perceived needs and an encouragement towards emotional dependence with the young child (particularly as an infant, where on-demand soothing and feeding, and sleeping with an adult may all be encouraged). In many more traditional non-Western cultures adolescence as a clear life stage with its own 'sub-culture' is not evident with physical labour, duties and responsibilities as well as an early introduction to spiritual life already apparent before the onset of puberty.

The more you examine how different cultures and the same culture over time view 'normal' childhood, the more difficult it becomes to know what is meant by a normal childhood. This means that there can be no universal way of defining which behaviours, thoughts or emotional experiences should be considered as abnormal. These differences between cultures are not differences of detail. From societies that focus on the individual to those that focus on the family, from prolonged indulgence of the young to early independence, from the predominance of non-verbal communication to the dominance of the cognitive and verbal, from physical closeness to physical distance, from conformity to freedom of expression, from narrow expectations to complete tolerance, from a spiritual focus to scientific rationality, from expecting ambivalence to expecting conflict, from freedom of movement to close scrutiny, from gender-specific expectations to non-gender-specific expectations, from duty and responsibility to play and stimulation – which version is the normal? Which version is the universal healthy and natural childhood from which others have deviated? We cannot define what an abnormal, psychologically or psychiatrically disordered child is until we've worked out what a normal child should be like.

Summary

In this chapter I have argued that our understanding of childhood distress and children's mental health (including the scientific investigation of this) is shaped by the cultural beliefs of a society. These cultural beliefs are influenced by our value systems and these in turn influence the meaning we give to a problem and what we then do about it. I introduced the term 'social construction' to describe this process and, using examples from Western and non-Western cultural beliefs about children and child rearing, explained how our beliefs about what constitutes a 'normal' and 'abnormal' childhood are socially constructed.

Chapter 2
Childhood in today's world

Rates of diagnosis of psychiatric disorders and prescription of psychotropic medication to children have increased dramatically over recent years, accelerating sharply over the last decade in most Western countries and more globally, with children from as young as two being prescribed psychiatric medication in increasing numbers. For example, researchers analysing prescribing trends in nine countries between 2000 and 2002, found significant rises in the number of prescriptions for psychotropic drugs in children were evident in all countries – the lowest being in Germany where the increase was 13%, and the highest being in the UK where an increase of 68% was recorded.[1]

Of particular concern is the increase in rates of stimulant prescription to children. By 1996 over 6% of school-aged boys in America were taking stimulant medication with children as young as two being prescribed stimulants in increasing numbers.[2] In the UK prescriptions for stimulants have increased from about 6,000 prescriptions in 1994 to over 450,000 by 2004 a staggering 7,000+% rise in one decade.[3] Figures on the prescribing of 'heavy end' psychiatric drugs in the US, the antipsychotics – drugs that until recently were only used for severe mental illness in adults – showed that prescriptions of antipsychotics to the young had risen five-fold between 1995 an 2002 from about half a million outpatient prescriptions per year to about 2.5 million.[4] This dramatic change in child psychiatric practice has occurred (until recently) almost without the public noticing, despite the profound implications this holds, not only for those children diagnosed and medicated, but also for our cultural beliefs and practices around childhood and child rearing more generally.

The most reassuring reason for this change in practice is that it is the result of scientific breakthroughs leading to the discovery of previously unrecognised psychiatric diseases in the young and of new ways to treat these. In this version the noble scientist and doctor are breaking new frontiers lighting up some of the darkest mysteries about children's behaviour and thus bringing new hope for alleviating the suffering of millions of children and their families.

Unfortunately it is a more worrying scenario that is closer to the truth. There are currently no childhood psychiatric diagnoses whose existence in the objective physical world (beyond the subjective imagination of the diagnosing doctor) is not disputed (see Chapter 3). The classification system we use for categorising child psychiatric disorders did not develop as a result of new discoveries, but as a result of a change in the way we think about and categorise children's emotions and behaviour (in other word from a new social construction of childhood).

The diagnoses we use in child and adolescent psychiatry were literally voted into existence by committee members of the American Psychiatric Association, particularly in the early 1980s when new diagnostic categories where coined (such as ADHD and autistic spectrum disorder [ASD]). The invention (or if you have been following my line of argument from Chapter 1, I could say the social construction) of these new diagnoses came before there was any new 'scientific' evidence to support the proposal that these diagnoses represented distinct conditions that could be found in children in all cultures. The search for biological evidence to support these new concepts accelerated, with much time and money being ploughed into the effort to uncover the biological basis for these newly described conditions. Despite the spectacular failure to discover any reliably reproducible evidence that conditions such as ADHD, ASD, or childhood depression are the result of genetic, biochemical, developmental, or other brain abnormalities, this has not prevented a growing belief that these conditions are indeed the result of known abnormalities in the brain. In a further 'trick' of classification, behavioural disorders such as ADHD and ASD (both disproportionately diagnosed in boys) have been classified as 'neurodevelopmental' disorders (in other words disorders in the development of the nervous system). This has meant that many of the behavioural problems that children present with end up being dealt with by paediatricians (as opposed to child and adolescent mental health services) who are the usual speciality that deal with neurodevelopmental disorders and most of whom have little or no training in assessing the significance of, and intervening in, the broader context of the child (such as their emotions, families, schools, cultural background, peer relationships and so on).

With these new diagnoses being viewed as biological; biological 'treatments' in the form of medications soon followed. The result has been what I have called the 'McDonaldisation' of children's behaviour. Like fast food, recent practice came from the most aggressively consumerist society (USA), and feeds on people's desire for instant satisfaction and a 'quick fix', fits into a busy lifestyle, requires little engagement with the product, requires only the most superficial training, knowledge and understanding to produce the product, can help to 'groom' lifelong consumers for psycho-pharmaceuticals, and has the potential to produce immeasurable damage in the long term to both the individuals who consume these products as well as public health more generally.

Why the increase in psychiatric disorders in the young?

OK, I've staked my colours to the mast and explained in rather passionate terms where I stand on the issue of diagnosis and medication in child psychiatry. Current practice in child and adolescent psychiatry is, in my opinion, rooted in political and cultural processes and relies more on a particular social construction of childhood and the task of parenting than science. However, this leaves the question of why this particular way of viewing children and dealing with their problems has become so dominant.

In the rest of this chapter I want to make an attempt at understanding what might be behind this (to me) rather worrying trend. This does mean that I stray further into a more theoretical discussion, which may, at times, appear to have little direct relevance to whatever problem you are currently facing. I don't expect all readers to agree with the opinions I express, however, whether or not you agree with my analysis should not affect the usefulness of the rest of the book which is more practical in nature.

If this increase in labelling and medicating children isn't the result of any scientific breakthrough, could it be due to a change in the way we understand and categorise children's behaviour or because of a 'real' increase in the prevalence of certain behaviour problems amongst the young (or of course a mixture of both)? Attempting to shed light on these questions requires us to examine the cultural context in which this change has occurred. So it's time to complete the timeline on Western culture that I started in the last chapter. It's time to look at 'where we have got to' in our ideas, beliefs and practices with children in Western culture (Western culture, particularly North America, UK and Australia, being the cultures that have seen the most rapid expansion in the numbers of children being labelled with psychiatric disorders and medicated for this).

We know that the space of childhood has changed in contemporary Western culture. Well-documented changes include:

- family structure – which has seen the demise of the extended family, increase in separation and divorce, increase in working hours of parents, and a decrease in the amount of time parents spend with their children;

- family lifestyle – there has been an increase in mobility, decrease in 'rooted' communities, and an increasing pursuit of individual gratification;

- children's lifestyle – which has witnessed a decrease in the amount of exercise, changes in diet with increases in sugars and fat and a decrease in essential vitamins, minerals and fatty acids, the 'domestication' of childhood due to fears about the risks for children resulting in more indoor pursuits such as computers and TV;

- commercialisation of childhood – there has been an increase in consumer goods targeted at children and the creation of new commercial opportunities in childhood, for example with foods, the 'parenting' industry, and the pharmaceutical industry;

- the education system – now has a strong emphasis on academic performance and competing in national league tables.

These changes are occurring at a time when our standards for what we consider to be acceptable behaviour in the young and acceptable child-rearing methods are both narrowing. It is now harder than ever to be a 'normal' child or parent.

The problem of narcissism

Societies like the UK are struggling with increasing problems of alienation, antisocial behaviour, alcohol and drug misuse, bullying, violence, eating disorders, self-harm, behaviour disorders, and neglect of the young, to mention but a few.[5] I do not wish to romanticise other cultures' concepts of childhood and child rearing nor do I wish to minimise the enormity of the task of improving children's lives across the world, particularly in the context of an aggressive market-led globalisation, destabilised communities, and regional conflicts with all the devastation to family life this brings, and where some local cultural beliefs are clearly a major problem (like female infanticide). However, I wish to state firmly and confidently that amongst those more stable and rooted cultures across the world, sophisticated ideas on childhood and child rearing spanning millennia exist, with many anthropological and other studies suggesting that such communities do not share the same magnitude of problems with antisocial behaviour, anxiety states and so on, amongst the young.[6] I am not saying that we can import sets of beliefs and practices from other cultures and simply transplant them here in Britain and expect them to work. However, some reflection on the nature of beliefs, values and practices in our own and other societies may help inform us about things that we can do in our bid to develop these in a way that can be applied to the unique British context.

In a small book such as this I cannot possibly explore in any detail the impact of changes in the space of childhood in Western modernity that I listed above. Instead I will limit myself to talking about the impact of a particular aspect of our value system that I believe has had a pervasive and negative effect on families and the sense of emotional security and well-being of children. This is the problem of 'narcissism'.

Narcissism describes the character trait of 'self-love' or in the more everyday sense 'looking after number one'. Narcissism has become a core value in modern life in consumer-orientated 'aggressively' capitalist countries. The spread of narcissism has, I believe, left many of our children in a psychological vacuum, preoccupied with issues of psychological survival and lacking a sense of the emotional security that comes through feeling you are valued just for being and have an enduring sense of belonging.

Let me attempt the difficult task of explaining why narcissism as a dominant value system may cause this. One of the dominant themes used by advocates of what is sometimes referred to as 'neo-liberal' free-market economy ideology is that of 'freedom'. At the economic level this is a core requirement of free-market ideology. Companies must be as free from regulation as possible, to concentrate on competing with others, with maximising of profits the most visible sign of success. There is little to gain from social responsibility (only if it increases your 'market share'). At the emotional level the appeal to freedom can be understood as an appeal to rid us of the restrictions imposed by authority (such as parents, communities and governments).

By implication this privileges a value system built around the idea of looking after the *wants* (not needs) of the individual (in other words narcissism). Taking this a step further, once the individual is freed from authority they are (in fantasy at least) free to pursue their own individual desires, free from the impingements, infringements and limitations that other people represent. The effect of this on society is to 'atomise' the individual into private spaces to the degree where obligations to others and harmony with the wider community become obstacles rather than objectives. In this 'look after number one' value system, other individuals are there to be competed against as they too chase after their personal desires.

This shift to a more individualistic and narcissistic culture and identity was recognised as early as the mid-1950s in America by commentators who began to speak about how the new 'fun-based morality' was privileging fun over responsibility resulting in having fun becoming 'obligatory' (the cultural message becoming that you should be ashamed if you weren't having fun, as there must be something wrong with you!).[7] With the increase in new possibilities for excitement being presented, experiencing intense excitement was becoming more difficult, thus creating a constant pressure to push back the boundaries of acceptable and desirable experiences and lifestyles, opening the doors, amongst other things, to sub-cultures comfortable with drinking to excess, violence, sexual promiscuity, and drug taking.

In this value system where others become objects to be used and manipulated for personal goals, social exchanges become difficult to trust as the better you are at manipulating others the more financial (and other narcissistic) rewards you will get. Such a value system, which ultimately seeks to eradicate or at least minimise social conscience, cannot sustain itself without our moral conscience beginning to feel guilty.[8] This is a basic psychological principle – if your happiness and satisfaction is gained through making others suffer, sooner or later you feel guilty. Thus it is no coincidence that those who are the most vocal advocates of free-market ideology tend also to advocate the most aggressive and punitive forms of social control. Whereas some of the resulting guilt-induced policy proposals are aimed at putting some restraint on unfettered competitiveness, greed and self-seeking; amongst those more fanatical believers in the ability of market ideology to solve its own problems (and thus best to leave the market to get on with it), the most common defence used to try and deal with the anxiety produced by this guilt is through finding target scapegoats for this anxiety. In other words, instead of facing up to the suffering the encouragement of narcissism brings to the world, our leaders need to convince us that our problems are due to other evils (like fundamentalist Islam, asylum seekers, homosexuals, single parents, bad genes etc.).

As a result another hallmark of Western culture's increasing psychological reliance on narcissistic impulses that encourage the avoidance of taking responsibility for its beliefs and practices is the so-called 'blame culture', which fills the media and contemporary culture more generally. We are, to coin a well-worn phrase, 'tough on crime/mental health', but getting nowhere with the 'causes of crime/poor mental health'. We build more prisons and employ more psychiatrists – a sure sign that despite best intentions, our approach to 'causes' is at best naïve, at worst a part of the problem.

With narcissistic goals of self-fulfilment, gratification and competitive manipulation of relationships so prominent, it becomes easier to see why so-called narcissistic disorders (such as antisocial behaviour, substance misuse, and eating disorders) are on the increase. Whilst I realise some of this argument may be hard to follow, I hope you can stick with it even though it is just one aspect of many that I am covering and even though talking about the general 'state of things' doesn't tell you much about any individual child or family. However, understanding what values guide our current 'social constructions' of childhood can tell you about the 'unwritten' rules that guide some of our behaviour towards each other, and help give some background knowledge that is useful when it comes to examining the scientific evidence presented in the next two chapters.

The effect on children

Our ideas about children, their behaviour, and how to deal with their problems, are shaped by the cultural situation. As a child in Iraq I grew up in a family-orientated culture. My childhood revolved around extended family. There was a group of women who looked after the needs of all their children collectively. When I needed a tonsillectomy when I was 10 years old it was arranged that one of my cousins would have the operation on the same day. My mother and her mother slept on mattresses on the hospital floor next to our beds while we recovered. Adults didn't play with us, we had a constant supply of other children to do that, instead they showered us with affection and called me 'champion of the world' when I insisted on this. There were no rewards for good behaviour. If I were 'naughty' my father would smack me or affection would be withdrawn. At primary school every teacher had a ruler at the front of their class, which would be used at the slightest sign of disobedience or disrespect. At play time the deputy head 'policed' the playground by walking around, holding a thick ruler in her hand and making it clear that minor indiscretions were not tolerated. I learned a clear hierarchy – that kindness and help should always be given to those younger than you and respect and obedience to those older. It is important to state that I am not making a value judgement at this point about whether these practices were good or bad (indeed in my own life as a parent I avoid the use of corporal punishment for moral reasons and because I don't think it works). What I hope you can see, however, is that different cultural realities produce different childhoods.

The attention given to individual cases of child abusers who society can disown as not belonging to or being (at least in part) the product of our culture masks Western governments' implementation of national and international policies that place children at great risk and the extent to which we may have developed, through the importance of 'narcissism', a culture that is essentially neglectful of children. For example, monetarist policies of the 1980s and 90s cut health, social, welfare and education programmes as well as enforcing similar austerity measures on developing countries, policies that had and continue to have particularly adverse effects on children and families.[9] A word of caution is important here. As I suggested in Chapter 1, making broad generalisations about any culture risks stereotyping. Thus while I think it useful to analyse some of the broad cultural trends found in modern Western societies, it is not all 'bad'. Uncovering and bringing to the public's attention the secretive world of child abuse has been a very important development in helping protect children. It is also worth acknowledging that some governments, including the current Labour government in the UK, have tried to address some of these issues with policies aimed at reducing the extent of childhood poverty.

There has also been a class-specific characteristic, with the plight of poor children being viewed as self-inflicted and the more insidious problem of neglect of children in middle-class environments often passing unnoticed.[10] With the increase in the number of divorces and families with two working parents, fathers and mothers are around their children for less of the day. A generation of 'home-aloners' is growing up. The amount of time children have with their parents has dropped dramatically in recent decades, and the back-up systems that extended families provided is dwindling. As families get smaller and spend less time with each other children lose the learning opportunities that are found in family-orientated social systems that are more geared to social responsibility (like the example of growing up in Iraq I briefly described above). Instead of having to negotiate several relationships within regular contacts with multiple kin, we increasing live in more emotionally charged small units trying to psychologically survive within a fiercely competitive and individualistic culture.

Children are cultured into this value system by virtue of living within its institutions and being exposed daily to its values. Ultimately reliance on aggressive free-market-style narcissism creates a system of winners and losers, a kind of survival of the fittest where compassion and concern for social harmony contradicts the basic goal of the value system. As this system is showing itself to be bad for children's happiness,[11] a similar process to the one which originated 'blame culture' (see above) works to try and distance us from the anxiety arising from the guilt thus produced. Instead of asking ourselves painful questions about the role we may be playing in producing this unhappiness, we can view our children's difficulties as being the result of biological diseases that require medical treatment (we can blame their genes).

These social dynamics also get projected directly onto children. Children come to be viewed as both victims (through adults using and manipulating them for their own gratification) and potentially 'evil' scapegoats (as if it is these nasty, out-of-control children's bad behaviour that is causing so many of our social problems).[12] This reflects an ambivalence that exists toward children in the West. With adults busily pursuing the goals of self-realisation and self-expression (these being the polite middle-class versions of self-gratification or as I am calling it – narcissism), having absorbed the free-market ethic, children when they come along 'get in the way' to some degree. A human being, who is utterly dependent on others, will cause a rupture in the Western value system goals of narcissism that individuals who have grown up in these societies will have been influenced by to a greater or lesser degree. Children cannot be welcomed into the world in an ordinary and seamless way. They will make the dominant goals of modern life more difficult. They will to some degree be a burden. Please note that this line of argument is not aimed at individual parents, quite the opposite. Just like blaming the child's genes is an easy way out, we also blame parents just as easily, making them responsible for children's criminality, poor behaviour and so on. No, this line of argument is about the way our value system affects the cultural attitudes and 'ways of doing things' which surround our and our children's lives.

I am aware in discussing this of the danger of slipping into a romanticised stereotyped view of childhood. This is an ever-present danger whenever we talk about childhood, as children are so often receptacles for the projections of our own unfulfilled wishes. Thus any conversation about 'the state of childhood' can easily become mixed up with sentiments about the general state of society. This also means that the current sense of 'moral panic' in many Western countries about the state of childhood is also likely, to some degree, to reflect a sense of 'moral panic' about where our culture is heading more generally. When we lament the loss of morality and lack of respect in the young and become worried about them falling victim to being attacked, exploited and 'losing out' we are simultaneously illuminating our own anxieties and concerns. If we are to create the 'cultural space' to have a proper constructive debate and a more reasoned understanding about how our culture influences children and our ideas about childhood then we must also address our own concerns as adults, otherwise we may end up colluding, without realising it, with our societies convenient use of children as scapegoats for its failings.

More and more surveillance

Thus far I have suggested that a basic feature of modern Western free-market-based culture is an increasingly narcissistic value system, which causes problems in children's and families' lives in a number of ways. I have outlined how we have developed an idea about the self that is shaped in a narcissistic direction, which then interacts with the collective guilt, fear of retribution, and fear of becoming a loser in the competition (or fear of pilfering of one's accumulated resources if you are a winner). This means that governments feel the need to police these potentially dangerous 'selves' in an increasing variety of ways. Thus, one feature that has also changed dramatically over the past century of Western society is the amount of surveillance to which parents and their children are subjected. The state has all sorts of mechanisms of surveillance and an 'army' of professionals tasked with monitoring and regulating family life as if they were aware that children are struggling in this culture and deal with their guilt by individualising the problem.

This is not to say that we do not need surveillance, as the effects of child abuse are many and far reaching. But we must also ask the question of what the impact of this is on non-abusive families (the vast majority of course). The increase in levels of anxiety amongst parents who may fear the consequences of their actions has reached the point where the fear is that any influence that is discernible may be viewed as undue influence, making it more likely that parents will leave essential socialising and guidance to the 'expertise' of professionals.[13]

Life has thus also become difficult for parents who are caught in a double pressure when it comes to raising their children. On the one hand there are increased expectations for children to show restraint and self-control from an early age, on the other there is considerable social fear in parents generated by a culture of children's rights that often pathologises normal, well-intentioned parents' attempts to discipline their children. Parents are left fearing a visit from Social Services and the whole area of discipline becomes loaded with anxiety. This argument holds equally true for schools. Parents often criticise schools for lack of discipline. Schools often criticise parents for lack of discipline. This creates a double pressure, which has resulted in more 'narcissistic' power going to children. Parents are being given the message that their children are more like adults and

30

should always be talked to, reasoned with, allowed to make choices, to express themselves and so on.[14]

This atomisation of society (making society more like a collection of competing individuals than groups of people with common interests and solidarity) also means that there is a lack of common ownership of rules and values with regard to the upbringing of children. Children may learn that only certain individuals have any right to make demands and have expectations with regard to their behaviour and with the task of parenting coming to be viewed in Western culture as one that needs childcare experts' advice in order to get it right, a form of 'cognitive parenting' has arisen whereby parents are encouraged to always give explanation and avoid conflicts. This hands-off, particularly verbal model of parenting is both more taxing and less congruent with children's more action-based view of the world.

Into this anxiety-loaded, narcissistically pre-determined vision of childhood and practices of child rearing, new diagnoses (such as childhood depression, ADHD, Asperger's syndrome) appear to provide a temporary relief to the beleaguered, intensely monitored child carers (nearly always the mother). By viewing children's poor behaviour and distressed emotional state as being caused by an 'illness', all are apparently spared from further scrutiny. The result however, fits into another aspect of our 'fast culture'. With the widespread application of the techniques of medicine to manage our children's behaviour and emotional state, particularly through the use of drugs, we have achieved what I call the 'McDonaldisation' of children's mental health, which I mentioned above.

It is only within such a cultural situation that these new disorders could have emerged out of the psychiatric imagination and then become popularised. They could not have been 'discovered' in cultures who were not plagued with anxiety about children's behaviour and parenting practices. In such cultures, institutions (like child and adolescent mental health services, psychological services, social services, etc.) whose task it is to survey and control children and their parents' behaviour, have simply not come into existence in the same magnitude. Thus it is no accident that over 90% of prescriptions of many of the drugs prescribed for childhood psychiatric disorders are prescribed within the economically developed West – although worryingly globalisation is helping export these Western practices, and so prescribing of these drugs outside of the West is increasing. And so it is to globalisation that I now turn.

Globalisation

Globalisation refers to the ever-increasing abundance of global connections. This 'compression of the world' has led to an intensification of consciousness of the world and a shortening of distance and time across the globe. Many forces have been at play to bring about the globalisation we are so familiar with today, including the extension of world capitalist economy, industrialisation, increasing surveillance (most notable through global information systems) and the new world military order. Global economic recession has also played a vital role as it spurred on a renewed globalisation of world economic activity involving the speeding up of production and consumption turnover. Another effect of globalisation is that over the last 35 years the volume of global migration has doubled. There is hardly a society left that can call itself 'monocultural'. Providing adequate services for populations who may have differing spiritual and cosmological beliefs as well as lifestyles is thus something that no society can afford to ignore. Two types of globalisation are often spoken about; they are: globalisation from above and globalisation from below.

Globalisation from above

One important recent aspect of globalisation is the 'neo-colonial' character of the way the world economy has become organised (often referred to as neo-liberalism, and based around the free-market economic system that I discussed above). This economic system has resulted in glaring inequalities between the 'developed' and 'developing' worlds and, from a human rights perspective, it can be argued that the global economic system is guilty of gross human rights violations and bears a large responsibility for man-made problems, such as poverty, starvation, lack of health care, militarisation and regional conflicts.

A more subtle impact of the neo-liberal character of globalisation is the export of Western value systems to countries with value systems born out of different traditions. This can result in undermining the stability of traditional beliefs and practices in many communities, which have served their children well, at the same time as producing points of conflict, antagonism and contradiction as the merits of different value systems clash.[15] All too often these conflicts are resolved in favour of the more powerful and influential culture (i.e., that of the industrialized West, which I argued above revolves around a narcissistic value system).

With regard to visions of childhood, it is not only modern Western citizens who Western professionals and governments feel should have a particular sort of childhood, but also worldwide populations who are often viewed as in need of civilization and development (according to Western ideals). As particular concepts of 'normal' childhood are exported so are particular conceptions (or social constructs) of 'deviant' childhoods. The perception that many third-world children are living 'different' childhoods can then be interpreted by Westerners as local peculiarities and instances of backwardness and under-development thus justifying continued efforts to export Western visions of childhood around the world.[16]

Just as problematic notions of child rearing are being imposed on countries of the South (this refers to the poorer, less industrialised countries of the world, that are mainly found on the southern side of the planet), so too are problematic notions of child mental health problems. Market economies – needing to continually expand markets – have allowed drug companies to exploit new, vague and broadly defined childhood psychiatric diagnoses, resulting in a rapid increase in the amount of psychotropic medication being prescribed to children and adolescents in the West. Evidence is emerging that this trend is spreading to countries of the poorer South where growth in the prescribing of psychotropic medications to children is occurring.[17] Little research has been done on the safety and efficacy of psychotropic drugs in such children, and the evidence that we do have isn't encouraging (see Chapter 4). This suggests that the Western individualised biological/genetic conception of childhood mental health problems is spreading to the countries of the South and may be undermining more helpful indigenous belief systems.[18]

Globalisation from below

The politics of neo-liberal globalisation also creates opportunities and paradoxes. Thus, neither the economic or cultural flow in the globalised world has been all one way. Globalisation has arguably brought many aspects of non-Western cultures, from culinary to medicinal, and from spiritual to aesthetic, into the mainstream in the West. The exceptions to the usual flow of economic power can also be seen with the emergence of powerful regions such as those of the so-called 'tiger' economies of the Far East. In many of these economies, traditional social values were successfully imported into the workplace (such as loyalty and protection for workers in return for conformity and hard work for the company) which helped enhance their economies' competitiveness.

Not only does globalisation create the space and possibilities for reverse cultural flow and thus new emerging fusions of identities, beliefs and practices, but, in addition, globalisation can produce resistance and, in some cases, a rediscovery of the importance of certain aspects of traditional culture. For example, despite prolonged attempts at influencing public opinion in Arab Middle East and North Africa, attitudes have, if anything, hardened against Western value systems and there has been a move to reaffirm and strengthen the regional, Muslim, identity.[19] The rapid increase in exposure to global influences may indeed expose children and young people to conflict between contradictory values systems. This conflict can lead to vulnerability and mental health problems, but it can also lead to innovative solutions, and new cross-cultural identities both within the 'outsider' culture and the young of the host community.[20]

Ideas on child development have long-established theories and practices in many non-Western traditions. These often emphasise growth of responsibilities as well as rights and see the basic social unit as the family and not the individual. Our lack of engagement with these cross-cultural perspectives represents a rather hidden form of institutionalised racism (or more accurately, institutionalised cultural hegemony) that has infected Western academic and political endeavours for a long time. Not only does this present real dangers to the traditions and knowledge bases in existence in the non-Western world but it means that, in addition, the populations in the Western world are being denied the opportunity to benefit from the positive effects that embracing non-Western knowledge, values and practices may bring.

Thus we have a situation where Western narcissism has resulted in Western children leading lives of material richness but with relative emotional and spiritual poverty, whereas the vast majority of the world's children live in conditions of material deprivation but with arguably greater emotional and spiritual richness. Globalisation means that these more 'traditional' family forms and childhood experiences are under threat as the West tries to impose its values on the rest of the world, at the same time as creating new opportunities for us to learn from other cultures.

Summary

In this chapter I presented some figures illustrating that there has been a rapid increase in the prescription of psychiatric drugs to the young. I suggested that this could be interpreted as a symptom of a 'dysfunctional' culture rather than due to scientific progress uncovering previously unrecognised disorders and treating them. I discussed a number of recent cultural changes that have affected children and explored the impact that a narcissistic value system has on children and families. I briefly explored globalisation, seeing in it threats and new risks for children and families but also new opportunities for positive learning.

Chapter 3
Common diagnoses

Sixteen-year-old Danielle was referred by her GP because the GP thought that Danielle was clinically depressed. My training taught me how to confirm this diagnosis. After listening to Danielle's story, I ask Danielle questions to find out what symptoms she presents with. She tells me about the trouble she has sleeping, how she is feeling low, hopeless and irritable and is often tearful. Danielle's mother confirms these symptoms and tells me about a family history of depression and how she (Danielle's mum) was currently taking antidepressants. I administer a depression-screening questionnaire and find that Danielle scores above the threshold for a diagnosis, thus 'confirming' that Danielle is suffering from clinical depression. I can now 'prescribe' some cognitive behavioural therapy adding an antidepressant at a later stage if necessary. By following such a format I provide the expert opinion that I was trained to provide and the whole session can be experienced (by me at least) as neat, tidy, contained, and easy on the emotions, if a little sterile.

By diagnosing clinical depression, had I discovered the cause or meaning of Danielle's current problems? Did I have any physical, objective evidence to back my diagnosis? The answer to both questions is no. Without physical evidence the diagnosis is based on my subjective belief (as passed on to me by my professional training), therefore far from discovering the cause or meaning of Danielle's problems I had *created* a new meaning for them – a story to explain the story she and her mother gave me. When I administered the depression questionnaire I created another story about my story about her story – that this questionnaire objectively measures something called depression. This questionnaire claims to have validity and reliability from being 'tested' on samples of depressed subjects – another story saying that this questionnaire has been adequately tested to prove that it measures what it is supposed to measure. I could go on to talk about the literature on reliability and validity, the different sorts of reliability and validity there are, how useful each is and what they each mean – a story about a story about a story about my story about her story. With each layer of story I move one step further away from Danielle's original story.

This is the reality for nearly all psychiatric diagnoses. There is no state-of-the-art rocket science going on here, merely that psychiatry, being a branch of the high-status medical profession, is allowed the cultural privilege to successfully claim that its own brand of mysticism represents a scientific truth. However, this particular brand of 'science', as in the case above, distances the doctor from trying to make sense of what has actually been happening in Danielle and her family's lives. Instead it imposes a more medicalised view that sees the problem as residing 'in' Danielle (rather than the circumstances she's found herself in) and can result in her and her family losing sight of their own abilities and becoming unnecessarily dependent on the 'expertise' of the doctor to 'cure' her 'illness'.

There are other ways to approach mental health problems. So my first meeting with Danielle and her mother didn't follow the above script. I listened to their story in a different way, framing my questions to find out more about the wider context of their lives, about important relationships, about current social circumstances, as well as positives and existing strengths.

I found out they had been living with Danielle's maternal grandparents after Danielle's mother and stepfather's separation. I found out that Danielle misses her natural father whom she has not seen for several years and that she never accepted her stepfather. I found out that one of the reasons for Danielle's mother and stepfather separating was because her mum felt guilty about marrying Danielle's stepfather, fearing this had a negative effect on Danielle. I found out that recently Danielle's mum had been seeing the stepfather and they were talking about getting back together. I watched Danielle give her mum the 'if looks could kill' look. I suggested we have a meeting with the stepfather. Mum agreed, Danielle didn't. More negotiation, and so it went on. The session felt messy, full of painful and complicated emotions, at times uncontained; but alive, engaged, and to me, more ordinary, real, and human.

In the previous chapters I have explained how we socially construct culturally developed ideas such as what makes a normal child and normal parenting. Now it is time to introduce you to a few key and common diagnoses used in childhood and adolescence. If you have read the previous chapters, you will realise that I believe that because we socially construct what makes a normal child and adolescent we also socially construct what makes an abnormal one. Thus we socially construct child and adolescent diagnoses.

When it comes to any individual child this is easy to demonstrate. All you need to do is ask the person making the diagnosis what test they have done on that child to confirm the diagnosis. After all there are no blood tests, x-rays or brain scans that exist that can demonstrate something wrong physically in the child. As a result so-called 'tests' for childhood psychiatric disorders are pencil and paper exercises, where a care giver is asked a series of questions about their child or asked to fill in a questionnaire. All such a 'test' can measure is that care giver's perception about that child at that moment in time. Whilst this is of course valuable information, it hardly amounts to a 'medical' test. It cannot measure something intrinsic in the child and would never be accepted as a valid basis for confirming a diagnosis in the rest of medicine.

What follows then is a brief introduction to how three common conditions are viewed in current practice (ADHD, autism and childhood depression), followed by a brief critique of this. Space hasn't allowed me to elaborate on other diagnoses such as obsessive compulsive disorder, conduct disorder, attachment disorder, bi-polar disorder, eating disorders and anxiety disorders, but similar critiques are applicable to each. Due to lack of space I have not entered into a discussion about the physical consequences of distress or the effects of physical disease on a young person's emotional well-being. It is also worth bearing in mind that my critique of the diagnoses we use does not mean that we should not manage, treat or otherwise help children who present with various forms of distress, far from it. Some, such as eating disorders, cause life-threatening physical problems that require life-saving medical and psychological treatment. My critique is simply to make the point that current diagnostic categories used in child psychiatry tell you very little about cause, treatment or outcome. This doesn't mean that child psychiatric diagnoses aren't useful for some people and in certain circumstances, but it does mean that these diagnoses should be viewed as a metaphor – a social construct (sometimes useful, sometimes not) – rather than a concrete entity that a person 'has', like diagnoses in the rest of medicine. In other words, whilst we can say someone who has been diagnosed with diabetes 'has' diabetes (and we can show physical test results that tell you the person's blood sugar is not properly controlled by the body), we cannot say someone 'has' ADHD (or show physical tests that tell you something physically abnormal is happening in that person's body/brain that is causing their behaviour problems). However, we may still choose to *describe* their behaviour as 'ADHD' for other reasons (for example, to communicate with others, for research purposes, to access particular services, etc.)

Attention Deficit Hyperactivity Disorder (ADHD)

The UK Royal College of Psychiatrists fact-sheet[1] on ADHD describes children with ADHD[2] as:

- restless, fidgety and overactive
- continuously chattering and interrupting people
- easily distracted and do not finish things
- inattentive and cannot concentrate on tasks
- impulsive, suddenly doing things without thinking first
- having difficulty waiting their turn in games, in conversation, or in a queue.

The formal technical definition for ADHD can be found in the American Psychiatric Association's diagnostic textbook, *The Diagnostic and Statistical Manual (DSM-IV)*[3] now in its fourth edition. This defines ADHD as:

A) Either (1) or (2):
(1) Six (or more) of the following symptoms of *inattention* have persisted for at least 6 months to a degree that is maladaptive and inconsistent with developmental level;

Inattention

- often fails to give close attention to details or makes careless mistakes in schoolwork, work, or other activities
- often has difficulty sustaining attention in tasks or play activities
- often does not seem to listen when spoken to directly
- often does not follow through on instructions and fails to finish schoolwork, chores, or duties in the workplace (not due to oppositional behaviour or failure to understand instructions)
- often has difficulty organizing tasks and activities
- often avoids, dislikes, or is reluctant to engage in tasks that require sustained mental effort (such as schoolwork or homework)
- often loses things necessary for tasks or activities (e.g., toys, school assignments, pencils, books, or tools)
- is often easily distracted by extraneous stimuli
- is often forgetful in daily activities

(2) Six (or more) of the following symptoms of *hyperactivity-impulsivity* have persisted for at least 6 months to a degree that is maladaptive and inconsistent with developmental level:

Hyperactivity

- often fidgets with hands or feet or squirms in seat
- often leaves seat in classroom or in other situations in which remaining seated is expected
- often runs about or climbs excessively in situations in which it is inappropriate (in adolescents or adults, may be limited to subjective feelings of restlessness)
- often has difficulty playing or engaging in leisure activities quietly
- is often "on the go" or often acts as if "driven by a motor"
- often talks excessively

Impulsivity

• often blurts out answers before questions have been completed

• often has difficulty awaiting turn

• often interrupts or intrudes on others (e.g., butts into conversations or games)

(B) Some hyperactive-impulsive or inattentive symptoms that caused impairment were present before age 7 years.

(C) Some impairment from the symptoms is present in two or more settings (e.g., at school [or work] and at home).

(D) There must be clear evidence of clinically significant impairment in social, academic, or occupational functioning.

(E) The symptoms do not occur exclusively during the course of a Pervasive Developmental Disorder, Schizophrenia, or other Psychotic Disorder and are not better accounted for by another mental disorder (e.g., Mood Disorder, Anxiety Disorder, Dissociative Disorder, or Personality Disorder).

Those with a critical eye would have spotted that words such as 'often', 'seems', 'difficulties', 'reluctant', 'easily', 'quietly', and 'excessively' that are used to 'define' ADHD symptoms are hard to define. For example, the word 'often' appears in every one of the above 'symptoms', but what does it mean? Does it mean that the child does those behaviours at least once a day or at least once a minute?

These lists of behaviours that are used to define ADHD appear in questionnaires that are then given (usually) to parents and teachers. These questionnaires are the closest we get to having a 'test' for ADHD. These questionnaires can only rate a particular adult's perception of a particular child at a particular moment in time and in a particular setting. In other words they are measures of the *subjective* perception of the adult filling in the rating scale. What they cannot be is an *objective* factual piece of 'hard data' that measures something intrinsic to the child.

There are no medical tests for ADHD. There are no specific brain functioning tests for ADHD. There are no specific psychological tests for ADHD. There are no specific observational tests for ADHD. A doctor, through that doctor's assessment of a child's history and reported behaviour problems, makes a diagnosis of ADHD. As mentioned above, rating scales, which the child's parents or carers and teachers fill in about the child concerned, are frequently used to assist the doctor when they are assessing a child for ADHD.

These days when making a diagnosis of ADHD, the doctor doing the evaluation does not need to observe the behaviours of hyperactivity, impulsivity, or inattention in the child concerned during the assessment. Making the diagnosis is based on taking a history (to see if the behaviours, according to those giving the doctor the history, started early in a child's life, and to exclude any other medical reason that may be causing the behavioural problems) and evaluating a couple of rating questionnaires. It's not what you might call 'rocket science', and ultimately the making of the diagnosis (or not) rests on the beliefs of the doctor and how they interpret the history and questionnaires. It's an entirely subjective process.

Hyperactivity, impulsivity and poor concentration are behaviours that occur on a continuum. All children, particularly boys, will present with such behaviour in some settings at some point. I know this as a parent myself. They are not behaviours that would be interpreted as abnormal whenever they occur. Contrast this to a hallucination (such as hearing voices that are not there) or a delusion (a firmly held and unusual belief, such as that someone on TV is sending secret messages to you, which is unshakable despite little evidence to support it) which, in Western culture at least, are viewed as abnormal in most circumstances. (However, even with these symptoms that are psychiatrically categorised as 'psychotic' symptoms – in other words, symptoms of someone deemed to be out of touch with reality – it is not as straightforward as many believe. For example, it is now recognized that many otherwise healthy and socially well-functioning people sometimes hear voices.)[4]

Without any medical tests to establish which individual has a physical problem causing these behaviour problems, defining the cut-off between normal and ADHD is arrived at by an arbitrary decision. Those who have argued that ADHD does not exist as a real disorder often start by pointing this out. Because of this uncertainty about definition it is hardly surprising that epidemiological studies (studies that measure how many have a disorder) have produced very different prevalence rates for ADHD ranging from about 0.5% of school-age children to 26% of school-age children.[5]

ADHD studies have found three to five times more boys than girls qualify for the diagnosis (and something like five to ten times more boys than girls get prescribed medication for ADHD). This is very similar to the gender distribution found more generally in psychiatric disorders during the pre-adolescent years. This is mostly made up of 'behavioural disorders' like ADHD, conduct disorder, and oppositional defiant disorder. Why is it that the behaviour of boys is seen as a particular problem during the primary school years? This seemingly obvious question is rarely discussed in the psychiatric academic literature (though extensively in other academic circles such as sociology, anthropology and cultural studies).

What sort of brain problem are we attempting to categorise here? Is it that boys generally have bad genes compared to girls? Is it something to do with the normal biological differences between male and female genes? Is there an interaction between boys' behaviour and changes in social expectations regarding children's behaviour generally? Do social changes in family structure, lifestyles, teaching methods, classroom sizes, rates of violence, rates of substance misuse and so on have an effect on our perceptions and beliefs about boys' and girls' behaviour, or on their behaviour directly? Has life got harder for boys in some way? Has life got harder for parents trying to control normal boy behaviour? Are we still compelled to pay more attention to the behaviour of boys than that of girls, only now we medicalise this (studies show that adults in Western societies are usually more tolerant of hyperactivity in girls than in boys)?[6] Do changes in teaching methods and a predominance of female teachers have an effect on how we understand and deal with boys' behaviour? These and other social/cultural questions relating to ADHD are rarely discussed in the medical literature (although I do discuss them at length in my book, *Naughty Boys: Anti-social behaviour, ADHD and the role of culture*).

If ratings of hyperactivity, poor concentration and disruptiveness are subjective then it is likely that we will find large differences in the way these behaviours are viewed in different cultures. This is indeed what is found. One finding from many studies, for example, is an apparently high rate of ADHD in children from China and Hong Kong. In these studies nearly three times as many Chinese as English children were rated as 'hyperactive'. However, when the researchers came to examine the results more closely they found that it was Chinese doctors rating Chinese children as hyperactive and that these 'hyperactive' Chinese children would not have been rated as hyperactive by most English doctors. In fact they turned out to be a good deal less hyperactive than English children rated as 'hyperactive'.[7] One suggestion for this finding is that it may be due to the great importance of school success in Chinese culture leading to an intolerance of much lesser degrees of disruptive behaviour. Whatever the reasons, it demonstrates that defining behaviour as hyperactive and disruptive is highly dependent on how your culture interprets the significance of such behaviour. This is further confirmed when you look at clinical practice within a country, let alone between countries. For example, studies have found that the rate of diagnosis of ADHD varied by a factor of ten from county to county within the same state (in the United States).[8] More recent international epidemiological studies (studies that carry out a survey on a section of the population) have also found substantial differences in rates of ADHD according to *DSM-IV* criteria. For example, a study in the state of Goa in India found that only 0.2% of the sample of young people they surveyed qualified for the diagnosis (compared to 3–7% found in most epidemiological studies in Western countries).[9]

There is also a more complicated issue that we need to be aware of in any discussion about where to place the boundary when diagnosing ADHD. This relates to the concept of 'co-morbidity'. When psychiatrists talk about 'co-morbidity' they mean that more than one diagnosis can be given to any particular patient. In other words, a child diagnosed with ADHD may also have symptoms that mean they can be given another psychiatric diagnosis, for example an 'anxiety disorder'. In such a case this child would be said to have ADHD with 'co-morbid' anxiety disorder (or visa versa – an anxiety disorder with co-morbid ADHD). Numerous studies demonstrate the high frequency with which these supposedly separate child psychiatric disorders occur in individuals with ADHD. It is estimated that about half the children with ADHD can also be diagnosed with a conduct disorder, about half can also be diagnosed with an emotional disorder, about one-third can also be diagnosed with an anxiety disorder and another third with major depression. Co-morbidity is so widespread that *at least* three-quarters of ADHD diagnosed children will have at least one other diagnosable child psychiatric condition. What does this all mean?

Psychiatrists use co-morbidity as a way of trying to explain clinical reality when it does not appear to match the diagnostic categories that researchers use. It's a way of maintaining a fantasy that there is a natural, probably biological, boundary between psychiatric disorders, where no natural boundaries exist. Thus we have another problem of how to interpret the meaning of the evidence in ADHD. How many of the studies that we have on ADHD are actually telling us more about a co-morbid disorder than ADHD? How relevant to clinical practice are studies that have ruled out co-morbidity before studying the affected individuals, given that most children with ADHD that professionals like myself see in clinics will have at least one other co-morbid disorder? How relevant are guidelines on treating ADHD when little research is being done on such treatment's effects on co-morbid disorders? But perhaps most importantly does the high rate of co-morbidity suggest that ADHD is more useful as a concept to researchers than to clinicians, as in real-life situations straightforward, uncomplicated ADHD is rare? If this is the case then our current knowledge base on ADHD is close to useless (castles built on sand), and current practice (which rarely acknowledges co-morbidity, and when it does so seems unable to step back and see the 'big picture' and instead focuses on each diagnosis as if they are separate features of the child) seriously misguided.

Because of these problems about how to define ADHD, it is hard to know what to make of follow-up studies. For example, some studies that show a higher number of young people with ADHD have accidents when they are compared to those who don't have ADHD. This, in scientific terms, is known as an association; you cannot say that ADHD causes the sufferer to have more accidents, as another factor could explain both. For example, is it that the study has simply found that more boys have accidents than girls, or that it was a co-morbid condition (like conduct disorder) that is more responsible, or is it a totally unrelated factor responsible for both causing ADHD and accidents (such as learning difficulties, low self-esteem, stress in the family, poor diet, etc.)? We could also get stuck in a circular argument about ADHD, as you might decide to define ADHD at the point where there is enough of a percentage increase in accidents over the rest of children and then use that as your evidence that ADHD exists as a 'real' thing.

From a philosophical point of view this lack of objective tests, confusion on how define the cut-off point between normal and ADHD, cross-cultural differences, and high co-morbidity leaves the practice of diagnosing ADHD stuck in a philosophical whirlpool that goes something like this: What is causing this child's hyperactivity and poor concentration? Answer: ADHD. How do you know it's ADHD? Answer: Because they have poor concentration and are hyperactive. Of course you can say the same thing about all the other co-morbid diagnoses (like oppositional defiant disorder, conduct disorder and so on). It really is based on astonishingly sloppy and unscientific thinking.

To really confuse matters there is a long list of famous scientists (e.g., Albert Einstein and Isaac Newton), authors (e.g., Hans Christian Anderson and Lewis Carroll), inventors (e.g., Thomas Edison and Michael Faraday), artists (e.g., Leonardo da Vinci and Salvador Dali), politicians (e.g., Winston Churchill and Abraham Lincoln), actors (e.g., Sylvester Stallone and Steve McQueen), musicians (e.g., Ludwig van Beethoven and Ozzy Osbourne), sportsmen (e.g., Michael Jordan and Paul Gascoigne) and comedians (e.g., Billy Connolly and Jim Carrey) all said to have had (or to have) ADHD. The list is endless.[10] What does this mean? What sort of a 'disorder' is this if it is associated with such 'greatness'? If it is ADHD that has driven these people to 'think outside the box' and end up contributing so much to our culture, would 'treating' ADHD deprive us of the creativity and inspiration that such people bring, and send us, as a culture, into some sort of dull, homogenous middle ground? For many of the above famous names, their main issue as children was surviving the school system where they attracted labels like stupid, lazy and unteachable. If the problem here is not these individuals' innate abilities, but a mismatch between them and their schools, is it the kids or their schooling environments (or neither) that we should be changing?

A powerful myth exists that sees ADHD as being caused by irregularities in brain chemistry that is primarily genetic. It is argued that scientists have identified malfunctioning genes that disrupt communications between different cells in parts of the brain that are in charge of self-control and inhibition and that they have demonstrated an abnormality in the brains of children with ADHD. No other child psychiatric disorder has received more attention in biological research than ADHD. There are over thirty brain scan studies of children diagnosed with ADHD that have occurred over the past three decades. Taken together these studies have not uncovered a consistent abnormality and have suggested a wide variety of different brain structures as being involved. In none of these brain scan studies have the brains of the children diagnosed with ADHD been considered in any way clinically abnormal.

The most widely debated issue is whether any of the minor differences these studies have found between the brains of children diagnosed with ADHD and the normal controls were due to the medication most of the children diagnosed with ADHD in the studies were taking. After all, animal studies have found that taking stimulants can cause a long-lasting change in the brain biochemistry of rats. The one scientific way to address this question is for a study to be carried out where children who have never been exposed to medication and who are diagnosed with ADHD are compared to an age-matched control group.

In 2002 a group of researchers published a study that claimed to have done this.[11] This study included three groups: 49 children diagnosed with ADHD who had never received medication, 103 ADHD children who had received medication (although no information was given as to how much and for how long) and 139 'normal' children who made up the 'control group'. Thus the authors had an opportunity to make numerous comparisons between the three groups, the most important being between the unmedicated group and the control group. However, compared to the control group, the unmedicated ADHD group were two years younger, and were shorter and lighter. This meant that all the researchers managed to demonstrate in their comparison was that older children had bigger brains than younger ones! What the authors chose to highlight instead was that there was no significant difference between the brain sizes of the unmedicated group and the medicated group and this was then used to conclude that medication is not causing the difference found in the brain-scanning studies.

This is fraught with problems, particularly as they provide no detailed information with regards the medication profile of the medicated group. It remains the case that the simplest way to settle the argument is to compare the brains of an unmedicated group with an *age matched* control group (in other words comparing the brains of a group diagnosed with ADHD who have never had medication with a group of non-ADHD children who are of the same average age, height and weight), which was not done in this study. Interestingly, given the size of the control group it is still feasible for the authors to do this with their existing sample and they have been challenged to do just that (choose a more age-matched control group from a sub-sample of their existing control group and compare these to the unmedicated group), but thus far they have not done this. One has to wonder why.[12]

Consequently, after three decades and over thirty research

studies we are still waiting for the one type of study that would confirm or refute whether there are any structural or functional differences between the brains of children diagnosed with ADHD and otherwise normal children. However, even if such a study was to be done and show a definite difference, this still does not mean that an abnormality in the brain has been proven as the cause of ADHD-type behaviours.

It is well known that the brain, particularly the developing brain, is very sensitive during its growth to the environment it finds itself in. For example, we know that a person under stress is likely to produce higher levels of the hormone cortisone than a person who is not. Furthermore, there is evidence to suggest that high levels of cortisone occurring over many months and years can have a significant effect on brain growth and development, particularly in infancy when the brain is growing at its fastest. We also know that everyone develops at different rates and so what we might be seeing (if a statistically significant difference in the size of particular brain structures were indeed proven) is simply those who are developing slower, or later, than their age group or the effects on the developing brain of living in a stressful environment.[13]

The belief that ADHD is a genetic condition is another of those ideas that has developed as a result of supporters of the diagnosis, ignoring matters of context. If we take as our starting assumption that behaviour such as motor activity, attention and impulsivity are temperamental characteristics (in other words part of normal variation, like personality characteristics), then the evidence fits much better. Viewing these behaviours as temperamental characteristics as opposed to signs of a medical condition allows more attention to other factors. Research on children's temperament has shown that problems result from a mismatch between the child's temperament and their environment. Even children who are highly difficult temperamentally can become well adjusted behaviourally if their family and other social circumstances are supportive.[14] Indeed a difficult temperament (such as high levels of activity and low attention span) is a poor predictor of future problems at school, the best predictors being parents' and then schools' ability to cope. What the genetic studies may have been discovering is that the behaviours we call ADHD are inherited in much the same way as other personality traits; whether these behaviours come to be perceived as a problem is 'shaped' by social factors. In their international consensus statement on ADHD, Russell Barkley and other prominent ADHD researchers[15] virtually admit this, when they compare the genetics of ADHD to the genetics of height. Since when has height been considered a medical disorder? It is simply a biological characteristic that varies from one person and one family to another.

Genetic studies on children diagnosed with ADHD suffer from many other problems. The main source of the evidence said to support the idea that genes are responsible for ADHD come from the finding that identical twins have higher rates of ADHD than non-identical twins. Because identical twins share 100% of their genes whilst non-identical twins share about 50% of their genes, it is (falsely) concluded that the higher percentage of identical twins both having ADHD compared to non-identical twins is the result of genetics. Concluding that the higher rates of diagnosis in the twin of identical as opposed to non-identical twins is evidence of genetic transmission ignores the substantial psychological difference involved in being an identical as opposed to non-identical twin. For example, substantially more identical as opposed to non-identical twins report identity confusion and are more likely to be reared 'as a unit'. Similar methodological problems have been shown to occur in the two other main methods used to try and establish a genetic link – familial studies and studies of adopted children with ADHD. None of the methods used are able to disentangle environmental and psychological effects from biological/genetic ones. Thus, just as we cannot conclude that genetics has no role, we do not yet have the evidence to conclude genetics has any role to play whatsoever. Indeed, we now have a growing number of molecular genetic studies (where scientists try to locate particular genes that may 'cause' or contribute to causing ADHD) that have set out to search for ADHD genes but have yet to reliably find any. This would seem to be leading us to the conclusion that genetics have a minor (if any) role to play in ADHD.[16]

Childhood depression

The UK Royal College of Psychiatrists fact sheet[17] describes children and young people with depression as follows:

> Most people, children as well as adults, feel low or 'blue' occasionally. Feeling sad is a normal reaction to experiences that are stressful or upsetting.
>
> When these feelings go on and on, or dominate and interfere with your whole life, it can become an illness. This illness is called 'depression'. Depression probably affects one in every 200 children under 12 years old and two to three in every 100 teenagers.
>
> ### What are the signs of depression?
> • Being moody and irritable – easily upset, 'ratty' or tearful
> • Becoming withdrawn – avoiding friends, family and regular activities
> • Feeling guilty or bad, being self-critical and self-blaming – hating yourself
> • Feeling unhappy, miserable and lonely a lot of the time
> • Feeling hopeless and wanting to die
> • Finding it difficult to concentrate

- Not looking after your personal appearance
- Changes in sleep pattern: sleeping too little or too much
- Tiredness and lack of energy
- Changes in appetite
- Frequent minor health problems, such as headaches or stomach-aches
- Some people believe they are ugly, guilty and have done terrible things.

If you have all or most of these signs and have had them over a long period of time, it may mean that you are depressed. You may find it very difficult to talk about how you are feeling.

Technically clinicians rely on the criteria outlined for diagnosing adults. For example the criteria for adults found in the American Psychiatric Association's *DSM-IV* list nine criteria for a major depressive episode.[18] Simplified, they are:

- feeling depressed, sad, or melancholy most of the day, nearly every day

- the inability to experience pleasure or excitement even when doing activities that used to be pleasurable

- serious weight loss or weight gain in a short period of time

- sleeping too much, too little, or not well

- sluggish or jittery movements that are noticed by other people

- feeling tired and experiencing low motivation or loss of energy nearly every day

- feeling guilty a lot, feeling worthless, feeling inadequate

• having trouble thinking clearly, being unable to concentrate or make decisions

• feeling helpless and hopeless, having thoughts of death or suicide or having a plan for suicide

An adult must have at least five of these nine symptoms during a two-week period in order to be diagnosed with major depression. The symptoms must also be preventing a person from functioning well in daily life. The only comment found in the *DSM-IV* about children is that 'in children the depressed mood can be an irritable mood'. In other words angry outbursts or frequent temper tantrums can be classed as a symptom of childhood depression.

However, child psychiatrists have tried to expand the notion of childhood depression by arguing that depression in children presents with different and less specific symptoms than that in adults. For example, eminent child psychiatrist Professor Peter Hill suggests more non-specific symptoms such as irritability, running away from home, decline in schoolwork, and headaches are more indicative of childhood depression.[19]

However, as soon as we start casting a critical eye we encounter similar difficulties to that found above in ADHD. According to the current criteria, psychiatric co-morbidity in childhood depression is so high nearly every child can be diagnosed with at least one other psychiatric condition,[20] raising the same doubts as ADHD with regard the specificity of the construct. Despite awareness of the continuity between normal sadness and clinical depression, the diagnosis assumes that clinical depression exists as a category (rather than on a continuum). It is unclear, however, who decides where the cut-off mark is, and on what basis.

Furthermore, the categorical diagnosis bears only a slim

relationship with levels of psychosocial impairment (in other words the degrees to which symptoms are interfering in daily life). Many children below the threshold of diagnosis show higher levels of impairment than those above the threshold.[21] Similarly, a diagnosis of childhood depression is only weakly associated with suicide (stronger predictors include a history of aggression and the use of drugs or alcohol). With regards to genetics, separating environmental from biological factors in the family studies has been virtually impossible, particularly as children whose parents have depression are at risk of developing a wide range of psychiatric disorders.

Some have argued that the importance of diagnosing childhood depression is that having childhood depression predicts getting depression later as an adult.[22] However, follow-up studies of children deemed to have had 'major depressive disorders' have used dubious standards for diagnosing childhood and adult psychiatric disorders; have discovered high rates of co-morbidity (in childhood and adulthood); have been unable to differentiate biological factors from continuing social adversity; and have not taken into account the possible effects of any treatment received (such as continuing morbidity as a result of toxic side effects of drug treatment and the experience of psychosocial adversity and decreased self-worth arising from becoming a psychiatric patient).[23]

The major problem behind the concept of 'childhood depression' is that it led to the medicalisation of childhood unhappiness, which in turn resulted in antidepressants often becoming a first-line treatment. It was only relatively recently (in the late 1980s) that our understanding of childhood depression began a far-reaching transformation. Prior to this childhood depression was viewed as a very rare disorder, different to adult depression and not amenable to treatment with antidepressants. We now know that this change in practice was more the result of good marketing than good science as antidepressants have been found to be largely ineffective in the under-18s with the potential to cause serious side effects (more about that in Chapter 4).[24]

Autism and the autistic spectrum

Autism in both mainstream scientific and popular literature is presented as a *disorder* that will, ultimately, be known and rendered transparent through the ceaseless efforts of scientific authorities. Controversy about the 'existence' of autism is less obvious than that for ADHD or childhood depression, possibly because in the past this was a rare diagnosis reserved for individuals who were clearly impaired, usually with multiple problems including moderate to severe learning difficulties.

Autism is a behaviourally defined disorder, characterised by qualitative impairments in social communication, social interaction, and social imagination (often referred to as the core 'triad' of symptoms), with a restricted range of interests and often stereotyped repetitive behaviours and mannerisms. Sensory hyposensitivities or hypersensitivities to the environment (such as being hypersensitive to sound) are also said to be common features.

In *DSM-IV*, autism is classified as belonging to 'The Pervasive Developmental Disorders' (PDD).[25] There are five sub-categories listed under PDD:

- *Autistic Disorder,* see below.

- *Asperger's Syndrome,* relatively good verbal language, with milder non-verbal language problems, restricted range of interests and relatedness.

- *PDD-NOS (Not Otherwise Specified),* non-verbal language and other problems that do not meet the strict criteria for other PDD disorders.

- *Rett's Disorder,* rare neurodegenerative (degeneration of the nervous system) disorder of girls.

- *Childhood Disintegrative Disorder,* another rare neurodegenerative disorder.

In common practice, Rett's disorder, and childhood disintegrative disorder are considered very rare mainstream medical disorders and are not usually dealt with within services for autistic spectrum disorders.

The triad of symptoms that are thought to be indicative of *autism* are as follows:

- *Firstly*, an inability to engage in reciprocal social interaction. Some have suggested that the autistic child fails to develop a 'theory of mind' (a theory about what others are thinking or feeling), and so cannot imagine what other people may think or feel and thus they lack empathy. Humans, animals and objects are thus treated in the same way.

- *Secondly,* there are communication problems, both verbal and non-verbal. Rather than having a problem with spoken language per se, it is almost as if the autistic child cannot grasp the point of communication. The affected child may not babble, is often late to speak, and has difficulties in understanding what is said to them. This defect in understanding spoken speech may be almost total, or may be subtle and merely take the form of literal interpretation of language. If the autistic child does develop spoken language, then there is usually an abnormality in the way it is used. Echolalia (repeating back what someone has said word for word) can occur. Volume, pitch and tone of speech are often peculiar.

- *Thirdly,* there is evidence of restricted imagination and a desire for rigid routines. The autistic child may form strange attachments to certain everyday objects, such as pieces of plastic or stones, or become fascinated with flicking paper or running water from taps. An obsessive need for routine is often found with temper tantrums resulting from any small change in the usual pattern of their life.

Asperger's syndrome is now thought of as being a milder version of autism with milder versions of the above symptoms but often without any obvious language impairment. Thus Asperger's syndrome presents with impaired ability to utilize social cues such as body language, irony, or other 'subtexts' of communication; restricted socialisation; limited range of interests; 'concrete' thinking; oversensitivity to certain stimuli; and other unusual or 'odd' behaviours. Various degrees of autistic symptoms and Asperger's are now commonly referred to under the umbrella term *autistic spectrum disorder* (ASD) often now just abbreviated to 'autism'.

Because of this broadening of the concept of autism into a spectrum (ASD) that includes large numbers of individuals who do not have any obvious intellectual impairments but rather appear shy, withdrawn or socially clumsy, the days in which autism (in all its forms) was a rare disorder have long gone. The prevalence of this broad spectrum of autism is approximately 5 to 9 per 1000 (close to 1% of the population) with the National Autistic Society claiming there are 500,000 individuals with autism spectrum disorders in the UK.[26] Like ADHD and all other pre-adolescent psychiatric disorders it is three to four times more common in males than females.

Autism as a diagnostic category has come to exist not because of any scientific breakthrough (such as identifying a core biological pathology) but as a result of a change in the way we think about certain behaviours in children. For example, the search for the genes presumed to cause autism have thus far (just like with ADHD) come up empty. Psychiatric conditions such as autism are often referred to as 'complex disorders' precisely because of the failure to find genes, while (in a peculiar kind of circular logic) failures to find genes are themselves explained on the basis of the 'complex' nature of the condition. The presumed genetic basis of autism rests largely on the results of family and twin studies (where higher rates of both twins having autism are found in identical as opposed to non-identical twins). Although autism may be 'familial' (that is it appears to be more common in relatives of those diagnosed with 'autism' than those who aren't), the fact that families share a common environment as well as common genes means that no valid conclusions in support of genetics can be found from these studies. As I mentioned before, the twin method is no better at separating out environmental factors than are family studies because, as ample research has demonstrated, identical twins experience more similar environments than non-identical twins, as they are more likely to be treated in the same way. Furthermore, as the diagnostic boundaries have changed and widened, it has become increasingly difficult to compare studies, as many use different cut-off points for diagnosis. Autistic symptoms have also been shown to occur in those who have experienced severe psycho-social deprivation, such as the children of the infamous Romanian orphanages[27] suggesting that the current belief that autism is a purely biologically based disorder is too simplistic.

The circumstances that created the possibility of diagnosing a child as autistic are ultimately less rooted in the biology of those diagnosed than they are in the cultural practices and economy of the time. Prior to the advent of mass schooling at the turn of the twentieth century the standards for classifying individuals as disordered were much less developed, the standards of normality much broader, and the mechanisms for social and individual surveillance that we take for granted today simply did not exist. This change in the way we think about and therefore classify certain behaviours took a marked acceleration toward the end the last century resulting in what some call an 'epidemic' of autism by the beginning of this millennium.

Thus a distinct medical/psychiatric condition called autism could not have emerged until standards of normality had been formalised and narrowed and standards of paediatric screening extended to a child's earliest years so that children with ASD could be 'identified'. This is not to say that there haven't been people throughout history who have displayed the symptoms we now group and define as autism, but to remind the reader, that calling this autism is more the result of a 'trick' of classification, as opposed to being the result of new biological knowledge.

A few decades ago autism was thought of as a rare disorder estimated to occur in about 4 per 10,000 children[28] whereas now it is thought to affect nearly 1% of children.[29] This massive increase in what we now consider to be autism means that a young person with virtually no language and unable to carry out even the most basic self-care can receive the same *behaviourally* defined diagnosis as another young person who is articulate, goes to mainstream school, is academically capable, but struggles to make friends. It is obviously absurd to have a spectrum stretching from speechless residents of day centres who need constant care to Einstein (who has been retrospectively diagnosed as autistic). We might just as well replace the term 'autistic spectrum' with 'human spectrum'! Indeed, many of the symptoms identified by Leo Kanner (credited with first describing 'autism' in 1943) and Hans Asperger (credited with first describing 'Asperger's' in 1944) are no longer regarded as the primary symptoms that identify 'autistic' children. For example, we are no longer concerned about identifying 'flat affect' (a kind of lack of emotional expression) as vital – something that was observed and thought to be central by both Kanner and Asperger – with much more emphasis now being place on 'social communication'.[30]

There have also been significant changes in the gender distribution. In 1966 the ratio of males to females deemed suitable for a diagnosis of autism was less than 2 to 1.[31] It is now thought to be more in the region of 4 to 1. As mentioned earlier such a gender distribution is very similar to that found in the rest of pre-adolescent child psychiatry. Moving from a more specific gender distribution to the more common one suggests that as we have broadened the concept we moved away from a primarily biological disorder to one that chimes with a broader social and cultural concern about the behaviour of boys.

This medicalisation of difference has some worrying parallels with the eugenics movement. Underpinning the eugenics movement was the view that all manner of socially undesirable traits (including mental ill health) was the product of faulty genes and that to improve the health of society these faulty genes needed eliminating. One of the main factors that made the eugenic philosophy acceptable for such a long period was the fact that respected members of the public (doctors) were arguing that a whole array of social and psychological problems were the result of individuals having genetic disorders. Successfully medicalising such issues opened the door to the use of medical 'remedies' (such as sterilisation) to deal with these perceived societal ills and eventually to the gas chambers of Nazi Germany.

There are some worrying parallels to be found in the search for 'autistic' genes in order to pave the way for aborting foetuses that may carry such genes. It suggests that we may be witnessing the emergence of a new eugenics with humanity once again being divided on supposedly neurological lines. Such a simplistic conceptualisation may be attractive for governments, teachers, health professionals, some parents and individuals, however, it also serves to deflect attention from the political implications of going down such a route, and makes implicit value judgements about what should and shouldn't be considered valuable in human beings. One interesting result however, has been the development of a 'user' movement that sees autism as something positive and autistic 'rights' as being akin to rights for ethnic minorities or homosexuals.[32]

Looking at autism through a more cultural framework also reveals how many aspects of the construct is culture specific. For example, lack of eye contact is considered a prominent symptom of lack of social skills in autism; however, the Japanese are very wary about establishing eye contact with relative strangers or with seniors. Similarly in a study of the Gusii tribe in Kenya, it was observed that according to their traditions mothers must make a conscious effort not to make eye contact with their children as they believe it can cause 'over-stimulation' particularly in the early years of the child's life.[33] In many ancient cultures, reading and writing, even where they existed, were not as favoured as much by the wise as (the apparently autistic by today's standards) rote memorisation, which for sacred religious reasons could not deviate from the original even by as much as one word. In societies that value such things it is not hard to imagine that a person lacking ability in many other respects might be considered special and even holy for possessing such a unique ability. Indeed many autistic characteristics are not at all dissimilar to devoted religious lifestyles, for example, seeking solitude, vows of silence, non-materialistic values, lack of personal relationships, daily following of rituals and so on.

In conclusion then, perhaps the increasing problem of epidemic numbers of children in the West receiving diagnoses of autism is a symptom not of something 'wrong' that we should try and cure in the individual, but that it has, like other childhood psychiatric diagnoses, become a barometer pointing to something 'unhealthy' in the culture/society that invented this. In this respect we could do worse than learning from our apparently less 'developed' but more tolerant neighbours in the poorer south of the world.

Summary

In this chapter I have argued that childhood psychiatric diagnoses have little scientific evidence to support the idea that they represent physical disorders of the brain and nervous system. Using three increasingly common diagnoses (ADHD, autism, and childhood depression) as examples, I analysed some of the 'scientific' evidence from a critical point of view to conclude that these diagnoses (like other childhood psychiatric diagnoses but unlike proven physical conditions in the rest of medicine) tell you very little (possibly nothing) about the cause, treatment and outcome of any individual child's problems. There is little evidence to support the belief that diagnosis leads to treatments that improve the well-being of those diagnosed, or that a diagnosis is required in order to choose an effective treatment.

Common diagnoses

Chapter 4
Common treatments

Having discussed some of the evidence that should lead us to review the usefulness and appropriateness of the current diagnoses used in child psychiatry, I now want to discuss common treatments used for children's mental health problems. A disproportionate section of this chapter is devoted to examining medication. This is because there has been a rapid increase in the use of psychiatric medication in the young and so careful attention to the evidence base on the effectiveness and safety of this practice is needed.

Medication

Rates of diagnosis of psychiatric disorders in children and prescription of psychiatric medication to children have increased dramatically over recent decades, accelerating sharply over the last decade in most Western countries with children from as young as two being prescribed psychotropic medication in increasing numbers (see Chapter 2).

These changing prescribing habits are being heavily influenced by the pharmaceutical industry's marketing strategies.[1] By joining in an effort to convince parents, teachers, doctors and other adults with responsibilities for the care of children that the emotional and behavioural problems children suffer with (and how many of us who are parents can seriously say that we have not had times where we were pulling our hair out with frustration or worry at our children's behaviour?) are caused by 'chemical imbalances' in the brain, drug companies are aware that large markets can become accessible to their products. According to some, by promoting a line of argument and publicity that creates new diagnoses and talks about them as being 'under-diagnosed' and 'under-treated' we have reached the age of 'an ill for every pill',[2] where marketing has triumphed over science. Nowhere is this problem more obvious than in the prescription of (as I will explain) largely ineffective and potentially dangerous psychiatric drugs to children and adolescents.

The drug industry has grown in profitability and influence in past 20 years and is now second in size only to the arms industry in the US economy. It controls much of the research agenda and employs sophisticated marketing strategies. Commercial rather than scientific concerns become the dominant driving force behind innovation. Within a system of capitalist global markets, drug companies have little choice but to do whatever works to increase the sales of their drugs, regardless of the impact on health care. Thus the hard sell is an inevitable consequence of the way that drug companies make money. Without strict regulation (and even with it) we should not be surprised to discover that some professionals notice that such a 'rich' industry provides many opportunities for greater personal wealth, which is reflected in the proliferation of links between doctors and the industry.[3]

Drug industry money is now everywhere, to the point where career advancement is clearly enhanced by a relationship with a drug company. Research confirms that marketing practices do influence prescribing habits.[4] Drug company influence can be found at every level, making it almost impossible to escape. Links between the pharmaceutical industry and the UK Department of Health have become so intertwined that the public's health is being put at risk, a recent and highly critical report from a cross-party group of MPs concluded. The report cites multiple failings at the United Kingdom's drug regulatory body for not scrutinising thoroughly enough data from companies seeking licences for new drugs and for not monitoring side effects adequately. It also blames lax controls at the Department of Health for allowing pharmaceutical companies to have expanded influence over the public and the medical profession, which, they believe, has led to over-prescribing by doctors and an unhealthy reliance on medicines by the public.[5]

In recent years it has become apparent that drug companies are also using consumer lobbying groups to their advantage not only by (often secret) generous donations, but also by sometimes setting up patient groups themselves. For example, the main pro-medication consumer support group for ADHD in North America is CHADD – Children and Adults with Attention Deficit Hyperactivity Disorder. CHADD has long received substantial amounts from drug companies. Critics believe that CHADD's basic function has become that of promoting stimulant medications manufactured by its corporate donors (for example, pharmaceutical companies donated a total of $674,000 in the fiscal year 2002–2003). CHADD also produce a monthly magazine called *Attention!* which drug companies buy in the tens of thousands and then place them in doctors' offices.[6] In the UK, the main parent support group for ADHD is ADDISS – Attention Deficit Disorder Information and Support Service. They also receive significant funding from the pharmaceutical industry. For example, a recent educational campaign 'launched to support parents of children with ADHD' includes a glossy booklet on ADHD called '*Family Stress Points*' produced using an educational grant from a drug company.[7] This situation has made it increasingly difficult for professionals, parents and other carers (not to mention children) to obtain impartial advice about the risks and benefits of exposing children to psychiatric drugs.

There are three main classes of psychiatric drugs used in children and adolescents; they are: stimulants, antidepressants, and antipsychotics. I will discuss each of them next.

Stimulants
Common brand names include: Ritalin, Equasym, Concerta, Dexedrine, Adderall

The most common medications used in the treatment of ADHD are central nervous system stimulants containing methylphenidate, such as Ritalin. These stimulants are from the same chemical family as the street drugs speed and cocaine; hence all stimulants are potential drugs of abuse and categorised in the legal system as 'controlled drugs' (like heroin and methadone). Stimulants' effects are not limited to those children who are diagnosed with ADHD. Stimulants have the same cognitive and behavioural effects on otherwise normal children and children with other psychiatric diagnoses.

A beneficial effect beyond four weeks of treatment in children diagnosed with ADHD has not been demonstrated yet in what is considered 'the gold standard' for drug trials – the placebo-controlled double-blind trial. (This means comparing the active pill with an inactive 'sugar' pill, where those participating in the study and those studying them don't know whether they are taking the active or inactive pill.) There is no evidence that stimulants result in any long-term improvement in either behaviour or academic achievement, with articles reviewing the literature on treatment with stimulants concluding that a beneficial effect on ADHD symptoms beyond a few weeks of treatment has not been demonstrated.[8]

Stimulants have the potential to cause many side effects, including serious ones. Common side effects include poor appetite, weight loss, growth suppression, disturbed sleep, unhappiness, irritability, mood swings, confusion, obsessive-compulsive behaviours, stomach-aches, headaches, and dizziness. Less common, but serious, side effects include, explosive violent behaviour, a flattening of emotions, and psychosis. Established side effects of long-term administration of stimulants include heart disease, lowered self-esteem, suppression of creativity, learning difficulties, excessive repetition, deterioration in performance on complex tasks, and, occasionally, death due to the toxic effects of stimulants on the heart. In the past couple of years hardly a month goes by without new concerns emerging regarding the safety and efficacy of prescribing psychiatric drugs to the young, forcing the regulatory body, the Food and Drug Administration (FDA), in the USA to issue new labelling in 2006 that warns about the danger of stimulants (and the new non-stimulant ADHD drug 'Strattera') due to concerns about them causing suicidal ideation, heart attacks, strokes, sudden death and psychosis.[9]

Animal studies have found that giving stimulants to rats can cause a long-lasting change in the brain chemistry. There has been a dramatic increase in the number of children who are receiving stimulants in Western society. The majority of children who are prescribed stimulants will remain on them for many years and increasing numbers are continuing to take stimulants into their adulthood. We do not know the effects on the developing brain, or the long-term effects on the heart, of giving children stimulants for many years, due to a lack of long-term follow-up studies.

Stimulants are powerful amphetamine-like drugs with potentially addictive properties. Children become tolerant to its effect resulting in gradually increasing doses being given to children as years on a stimulant clock up. The potential for tolerance and addiction is further demonstrated by withdrawal states (known as the rebound effect, which presents as increased excitability, activity, talkativeness, irritability and insomnia) seen when the last dose of the day is wearing off or when the drug is withdrawn suddenly. Stories of adults becoming addicted to prescribed stimulants are becoming more common.

Research has focused almost exclusively on short-term outcomes. Why so little long-term studies from the manufacturers? The few long-term studies that have been completed (usually by looking at what is now happening in the lives of adults who were prescribed stimulants when they were young) have shown that stimulants do not appear to result in any long-term improvement in behaviour, relationships, or academic achievement.[10] Despite the lack of evidence for any longterm effectiveness, stimulants are usually prescribed continuously for seven, eight or more years, with children as young as two being prescribed the drug in increasing numbers despite the manufacturer's licence stating that it should not be prescribed to children under six.

In a world run by those with the power to 'buy' media attention, it is not uncommon for single studies to become the basis on which practice develops. One such study was a large multi-centre trial in the United States, testing the efficacy of methylphenidate (Ritalin) for children diagnosed with ADHD. This study is known as the MTA (Multimodal Treatment of ADHD) study and was first published in 1999.[11] I heard an eminent professor of child psychiatry in the UK state at a large conference attended by child psychiatrists and paediatricians shortly after the publication of the results of this trial, that the implication of this study is that we should be treating children diagnosed with ADHD with stimulant medication as the first line and possibly only treatment. It is notable that in the years since the publication and popularisation of this study there has been a sharp rise in the rates of stimulant prescription in the UK and the practice that professor was recommending has become the norm.

The MTA study was large (with over 400 children) and compared four groups of children who were given either: medication only; intensive behavioural therapy only; combined behavioural therapy and medication; or standard community care. The study lasted 14 months and concluded that the medication-only and combined behaviour therapy and medication groups had the best outcome, with the combined group having only a marginally better outcome than the medication-only group. A closer look inevitably brings up important questions of methodology as well as the question of a conflict of interest.[12] The principle investigators were well-known advocates of medication with long-established financial ties to the pharmaceutical industry. Methodologically this was not a placebo-controlled double-blind clinical trial (see above) and the parents and teachers who participated in the study were exposed to pro-drug propaganda at the start of the study, thus putting them in a mindset of positive expectation for change in those children receiving medication. Interestingly there was one group who rated symptoms through observing children in the classroom, and who were 'blind' to the treatment status of the children they were observing (in other words they didn't know which children were taking medication). These researchers found no difference between any of the treatment groups on the behavioural measures they were using. Not surprisingly this important finding was given no importance in the study conclusions. There are also many question marks with regard the selection and recruiting process, the behavioural interventions used, and the lack of attention to the number of children experiencing side effects. In addition, two-thirds of the 'standard community care' group were also receiving the same stimulant medication during the period of the study, yet were placed in the poorest outcome category. Finally, it is important to realise that the 'behaviour therapy' group had completed their therapy and had no further face-to-face contact with a doctor or therapist some four to six months before the trial ended, whilst those in the 'medication-only' group continued to receive regular and frequent face-to-face contact with a prescribing doctor right up until the end of the active study period at 14 months. Given that about two-thirds of the 'standard community care' group were also taking medication yet placed in the 'poorest' outcome group, one likely reason for the finding that participants in the 'medication-only' and 'combined medication and behaviour therapy' groups had the best outcome is because they received extra attention from doctors compared to the other groups (the placebo effect). If this were the case (rather than the better outcome being down to the medication) then we should expect that advantages of the medication groups are lost once the active treatment phase of the study is over. This is exactly what happened.

The participants in the above study were followed up again 10 months after the end of the study – in other words, after a total of 24 months since the start of the study.[13] These results are no longer looking so impressive. While the percentages of children with normalised symptom levels (in other words, those who, in the opinion of the researchers, were no longer displaying ADHD symptoms) were essentially unchanged for the behaviour therapy-only and community care groups, they had declined substantially for the combined and medication-only groups. The medication-only group now had a similar percentage to the behaviour therapy-only group. Furthermore, there was now no evidence of significant treatment group differences in social skills, reading achievement, and parents' use of negative/ineffective discipline strategies, and those who were receiving medication were now significantly physically shorter and lighter than those who were not.

Most recently the three-year outcome for the MTA study was published (a further year after the 24-month outcome study).[14] All the advantages with regard to symptoms of ADHD for the medication-only and combined medication/behaviour therapy groups had been lost, whilst the improvements in the behaviour therapy-only group had remained stable. Since the

73

end of the study (at 14 months) participants had been free to pursue whatever treatment they wanted. Some children had started medication and others on medication had stopped. The behaviour therapy group remained the group with the lowest use of medication. Furthermore when the researchers analysed outcomes for those who had used medication in the previous year they found that they had a worse outcome than those who hadn't. In addition, those who had higher use of medication also had higher rates of delinquency at three years, and they were significantly shorter (by an average of over 4 cm) and lighter (by an average of over 3 kg) than those who hadn't used medication. Thus the study that was loudly hailed across the media and within the medical profession, and has been repeatedly quoted including in Department of Health and National Institute for Health and Clinical Excellence (NICE) guidelines, as the study that demonstrated that stimulants should be used to treat ADHD, has conclusively discovered: (a) that stimulants are not more effective in the longer term than behaviour therapy and may indeed have a slightly worse outcome; (b) that stimulants cause significant and enduring side effects, placing question marks on their safety; and (c) that psychotherapeutic approaches (in this case behaviour therapy) are safer, just as effective and have beneficial effects that are more likely to be enduring.

Thus the scientific conclusion that we can make from analysing the evidence on treatment of ADHD with stimulants is that despite many studies, the evidence to support the idea that treatment with stimulants produces *long-lasting* benefits is absent. Indeed, according to Dr William Pelham, who was on the steering committee for the MTA studies, and who recently 'broke ranks' and spoke about the negative effects of drug company influence: '*No drug company in its literature mentions the fact that 40 years of research says there is no long-term benefit of medications* [for ADHD]. *That is something parents need to know.*'[15]

More difficult to assess are the possible social and cultural effects such widespread use of stimulants in children may have. Doctors may be unwittingly convincing children to control and manage themselves using medication, a pattern that may carry on into adulthood as the preferred or only way to cope with life's stresses. Clinically I have come across children on stimulants who have admitted that they were secretly self-medicating at times of stress. Parents, teachers and others may lose interest in understanding the meaning behind an ADHD-labelled child's behaviour beyond that of an illness internal to the child that needs medication.

Stimulants like Ritalin are also drugs of abuse as they can be crushed and snorted to produce a high. Surveys have shown that a significant proportion of adolescents in the United States self-report using Ritalin for non-medical purposes. Surveys have shown that between 3 and 16% of college students in the US admit to the use of non-prescribed stimulants. In addition, a significant proportion of those prescribed stimulants for ADHD have also been found to be either taking other stimulants in addition to their own, or to be misusing their prescribed medication.[16] The chemical effects of Ritalin on the brain are very similar to that of cocaine, which is one of the most addictive drugs, and cocaine users report that the effect of injected Ritalin is almost indistinguishable from that of cocaine.[17]

Studies on the likelihood of substance misuse amongst those with a diagnosis of ADHD treated with a stimulant often conclude that those treated with a stimulant are less likely to abuse substances when compared to those with ADHD who were not treated with stimulants. Whilst it is thankfully rare for children prescribed a stimulant which is taken by mouth to becoming physically 'addicted', an unanswered question remains as to whether taking stimulants as a child sensitises the brain toward future substance abuse. The largest community-based study examining this issue followed up nearly 500 children from the 1970s and right into their late twenties. They found a significant increase in amphetamine, cocaine and tobacco dependence amongst ADHD subjects who had taken stimulants when compared to 'untreated' controls. Furthermore they discovered a linear relationship between the amount of stimulant treatment and the likelihood of either tobacco or speed/cocaine dependence (in other words the more stimulant these young people had received over the years, the greater the likelihood of their becoming addicted to tobacco, speed or cocaine by their late twenties).[18]

Use of stimulants in children therefore remains a controversial issue for reasons that go well beyond its effectiveness and side effects. Yet this important information for parents, who are trying to make the difficult decision as to whether or not to agree to their children taking a stimulant, is information that is rarely given by prescribers.

Antidepressants
Common brand names: Prozac, Zoloft, Luvox, Paxil
The evidence is now clear with regard the use of antidepressants in childhood – they are no more effective (even in the short term) than a sugar pill (placebo) and have considerable dangers attached to their use, particularly related to them causing an increased risk of developing suicidal thoughts. Despite this, antidepressants remain widely prescribed to children and adolescents.

It is well established that the older tricyclic antidepressants (such as imipramine and amitryptyline) are not effective for childhood depression.[19] The evidence now clearly indicates that neither are the newer Selective Serotonin Reuptake Inhibitor (SSRI) antidepressants (such as Prozac and Zoloft). In 2004, Jureidini and his colleagues,[20] writing in the *British Medical Journal*, reported that none of the studies on SSRI antidepressants for childhood depression have, on measures relying on patient- or parent-reported outcomes, showed significant advantage over a placebo. No data regarding rates of self-harm, presentations to emergency or mental health services, or school attendance were presented in any of the studies they reviewed leading them to conclude that investigators exaggerated the benefits and downplayed the dangers of the newer antidepressants for children. A review published in another leading journal, the *Lancet*, the following week found that the pharmaceutical industry had been 'sitting on' many unpublished trials, which showed that newer antidepressants were even less effective and more harmful for children than suggested by the published trials.[21]

Despite this accumulating evidence about the lack of effectiveness and potential dangers of SSRI antidepressants, the UK National Institute for Health and Clinical Excellence (NICE) guidelines for depression in children and young people repeated an earlier UK Committee on the Safety of Medicines conclusion that there was still one antidepressant with a favourable balance of benefit over risk – fluoxetine (brand name: Prozac).[22] Given its similar pharmacological properties there is no theoretical reason why fluoxetine should achieve a significantly different profile than other SSRIs; and indeed it doesn't.

The Treatment of Adolescents with Depression Study (TADS)[23] is the most influential pro-fluoxetine study and provides a good example of how the publicity (of efficacy and safety in treating childhood depression) for this study does not match the published findings (let alone any undisclosed unpublished ones). Whilst the study was funded by a US government agency, investigators who had received significant industry funding conducted it. The investigators claimed to show an advantage for fluoxetine, especially when combined with cognitive-behaviour therapy (CBT). However there were flaws in the way they reported their data.[24] TADS include a double-blind comparison of fluoxetine against placebo and an unblinded comparison between CBT alone and fluoxetine with CBT (in other words participants who were in the CBT plus fluoxetine arm knew they were taking an antidepressant and may well have been discussing this in their therapy sessions; they also didn't have a group with CBT and placebo). This lack of patient-blinding and placebo-control in the latter two groups is likely to exaggerate the benefit seen in the fluoxetine with CBT group, who received more face-to-face contact and knew (as did their doctors) that they were not receiving a placebo. Furthermore the poor response of the CBT-alone group is a finding inconsistent with the rest of the psychotherapy outcome literature for childhood depression, raising questions about the quality of the psychotherapeutic intervention in this study. Comparing results across all four groups is therefore misleading. The one valid finding from TADS is the lack of a statistical advantage for fluoxetine over placebo on the primary measure the investigators used – in other words, just like other antidepressants in childhood studies, fluoxetine in this study is no more effective than a sugar pill. Despite the exclusion of known suicidal behaviour for anyone participating in the study, TADS found a trend to more suicidal behaviour (six attempts in the fluoxetine groups, versus one in the no-fluoxetine groups), consistent with other trials of SSRIs. Putting together that result with the lack of clinically significant advantage to drug over placebo and similar findings in the previous studies comparing fluoxetine and placebo,[25] the profile for fluoxetine is similar to all other SSRI antidepressants – it has little efficacy and is potentially dangerous.

One of the likely reasons for the continued and often routine use of antidepressants is the high placebo response found in the studies (in other words a large percentage of the children were getting better, even those just taking a sugar pill).

It is thus likely that many doctors see improvements after prescribing an antidepressant for a young person in distress and subsequently attribute improvements to the prescription. This high placebo response may thus reinforce a doctor's prescribing habits and it has been difficult for many doctors faced with a distressed young person to accept that SSRIs may be ineffective. On this point Professor Jane Garland, a participant in Sertraline (an SSRI) trials, but who later became sceptical about their methodology and reporting, writes 'The high placebo response of SSRIs may reinforce physician prescribing, and it has been difficult for many physicians to accept that SSRIs may be ineffective. A complicating factor is that the public at large has now accepted the model of depression as a chemical imbalance for which medication is the treatment of choice, and the physician may experience pressure to prescribe. The disappointing reality is that antidepressant medications have minimal to no effectiveness in childhood depression beyond a placebo effect.'[26]

Interestingly, if we look at the history of the use of antidepressants with children we find that child psychiatry as a profession had already endorsed the use of SSRI antidepressants to become a well-established part of daily practice long before any of the major studies in children were even published.[27] The scene was thus set for marketing spin to take precedence over scientific accuracy. As a result it appears that one reason for doing the studies in the first place was to justify already well-established prescribing patterns. It created a trend of 'because everyone else is doing it', which has become difficult to reverse despite the evidence. However, the evidence couldn't be clearer – antidepressants in children are ineffective and can be dangerous.

Antipsychotics

Common brand names: Risperdal, Zyprexia, Seroquel, Abilify

One of the most concerning trends is that of the increasing use of 'major tranquilisers' also called 'antipsychotics' for children displaying behaviour problems. These are powerful drugs traditionally used for adults suffering with what are considered 'severe' mental illnesses such as schizophrenia (although even here the evidence for the benefit is mixed at best, with much evidence showing that when antipsychotics are used for many years, they can cause subtle forms of brain damage, diabetes and other endocrine problems, and early death).[28] Its use for less severe psychiatric problems and for children is a relatively new and poorly evaluated phenomenon.

According to a report in 2006 in *USA Today,*[29] outpatient prescriptions of antipsychotics for children ages 2 to 18 in the USA leapt fivefold – from just under half a million to about 2.5 million – between 1995 to 2002. This figure doesn't include prescriptions at psychiatric hospitals or residential treatment centres. The majority of these prescriptions were for behavioural problems in children with diagnoses such as ADHD and 'bipolar disorder' (an increasingly popular diagnosis used in the young in the US, but not so commonly used in the UK).

A good example of the type of the misinformation that the medical community routinely receives comes from Susan Morgan and Eric Taylor's (who is regarded as one of the most eminent child psychiatrists in the UK) recent editorial in the *British Medical Journal* [30] (believed to be the medical journal with the highest readership worldwide). In their editorial entitled 'Antipsychotic drugs in children with autism' they appear to take a moderate stance suggesting that antipsychotic drugs should not be used indiscriminately in children with autism. However, having stated this they go on to argue that in the right circumstances antipsychotics should be used in children diagnosed with autism who are presenting with behavioural problems. They note that antipsychotics have not been licensed in the UK for this purpose (in other words the authorities who evaluate these drugs have not approved their use for behavioural problems in children with autism), however they state, 'We consider off label use [of antipsychotics] is justified when other approaches fail or are unfeasible'. This effectively leaves the door open for the continued increase in the use of (off-label) antipsychotics, as the reader is left to wonder what other approaches to use and for how long before deciding they have failed. Furthermore, 'unfeasibility' of other approaches is becoming a big issue as the increasing popularity of the diagnosis of autism (see Chapter 3), together with the diagnosis becoming more often than not the responsibility of busy community paediatricians, means 'other approaches' are thin on the ground. They further recommend 'Diagnosis should distinguish between aggression and other seriously challenging behaviours (which may justify an antipsychotic agent) and lesser levels of irritability (which may not).' However, they don't explain how a clinician is supposed to differentiate between what one should consider 'seriously' challenging behaviour and irritability. They also talk about autism as if this condition was an already unchallengeable, established fact of medicine, neglecting to mention that the boundaries of this condition have expanded rapidly in recent years (see Chapter 3). Much of the increase in diagnosis has been amongst non-learning disabled boys in mainstream schools who have a variety of behavioural difficulties. If, as I and many other critics contend, this is part of a socio-cultural trend of medicalising behaviour problems in response (at least in part) to an increasing sense of moral panic about children in general and boys in particular (see Chapters 1 and 2), then given that their advice is open to such broad interpretation, the outcome is likely to be an increase in the use of antipsychotics for managing challenging behaviour in the young.

But the real problem of this editorial is the lack of scientific support for their position. In support of their recommendation to use antipsychotics for challenging behaviour they refer to two studies [31] only, a far cry from the usual requirement of having several independent studies to compare. Most readers will simply accept at face value what Morgan and Taylor say about these two studies, which is that using an antipsychotic (in this case risperidone – brand name Resperdal) for behaviour problems in children diagnosed with autism appears to be safe and effective. However, a more critical review of these two studies reveals anything but encouraging news for this practice. Firstly, both studies were only eight weeks in duration, far off the many years that drugs prescribed to pacify behaviour are usually used for. Secondly, one of the studies reviewed their subjects at six months: this showed a familiar pattern seen with drug treatment for behavioural problems – that of diminishing returns, with less than half of the group that had received risperidone now rated as 'improved' (interestingly they do not provide the data for the placebo group outcome at six months). Thirdly, a decrease in challenging behaviour in those receiving an antipsychotic at a sufficient dose is really a foregone conclusion, after all antipsychotics are not classified as 'major tranquillisers' for nothing. Whether this is viewed as a therapeutic effect or side effect depends on your perspective. Reflecting this fact, both studies rated high levels of 'somnolence' (drowsiness or sleepiness) of around 70%. This leads to the rather peculiar scenario where arguably the same pharmacological effect is simultaneously rated as therapeutic (decrease in aggressive behaviours) and an adverse effect (somnolence).

What is more shocking is the minimising of serious adverse effects, which were prevalent in both studies. To give just one example: both studies found the group receiving risperidone put on more weight than the group with the placebo, in one this was an average of 2.7 versus 0.8 kg, and in the other this was an average of 2.7 versus 1.0 kg. Remember this was after only eight weeks. These drugs are 'heavy'-end psychiatric drugs with potentially serious consequences for a person's physical health including weight gain, diabetes, permanent movement disorders and heart problems. A *USA Today* study of data collected from 2000 to 2004 shows at least 45 deaths of children in which an antipsychotic was listed in the official Food and Drug Administration (FDA) database as the 'primary suspect'.[32] Bearing in mind that the FDA's Adverse Events Reporting System database is thought to capture only 1% to 10% of drug-induced side effects and deaths, this should be sufficient to cause considerable alarm about any proposal to recommend the use of these drugs with such meagre evidence.

Thus what the editorial reveals is that Morgan and Taylor are most certainly not the moderates they wish to present themselves as. Indeed they note that Janssen-Cilag (the drug company that makes Risperdal) withdrew their application for risperidone to be licensed in the UK for use in autism, due to fears about its safety. As a result they actually outdo a drug company in their keenness for use of psycho-pharmaceuticals in controlling children's behaviour and go on to suggest doctors should carry on using it for this (out of licence) indication. Their position only adds to the current social trend of using powerful, risky and largely ineffective medicines to control the behaviour of a group of citizens (children) who have never had a say in what is being imposed upon them and with scant evidence to back up the validity or utility of such practice. The lesson here is clear. As with many other areas of medicine we should not always trust what 'opinion leaders' say.

The above points about psychiatric medication for the young lead to the conclusion that overall, psychiatric drugs are not particularly effective and carry many dangers. As with my critique of diagnosis in the last chapter, this does not necessarily mean that psychiatric drugs should *never* be used in young people, but it does suggest that they are currently over-used. Young people and their parents should be enabled (through access to information such as the above) to challenge doctors to provide a clear rationale and evidence for using psychiatric medication, particularly if they feel unhappy about it being prescribed.

Psychotherapy

The good news is that unlike medication for children and adolescents, psychotherapeutic approaches have long established themselves as both safe and effective.[33] Furthermore, beneficial effects may be more enduring than with medication, given the increased likelihood of 'relapse' once the medication is stopped.

However, an important question that has been debated for decades is whether there are any particular advantages for particular techniques with particular problems (or diagnoses) as opposed to common factors with different psychotherapies being more important (in other words, psychotherapy in general being effective for psychiatric disorders with little advantage for one particular approach/method over another). This is sometimes referred to as the debate between the 'medical model' of psychotherapy (specific techniques have specific 'ingredients' that treat specific problems) and the 'contextual model' of psychotherapy (the 'common' factors to all psychotherapy being more important than specific techniques).

The evidence is now so overwhelming that the debate is pretty much settled. The 'contextual model' explains the research findings much better than the 'medical model'. All recognised formal psychotherapies (in otherwords where someone has been properly trained to deliver a particular technique) are effective to roughly the same degree, no matter what the psychiatric problem is.[34] Furthermore, decades of increasingly sophisticated research into treatment outcome for psychiatric disorders *has found little to support*: (a) the ability of psychiatric diagnosis in either selecting the course or predicting the outcome of therapy; (b) the superiority of any specific therapeutic approach over any other for any particular psychiatric problem; and (c) the superiority of pharmacological (medication) over psychotherapeutic treatment for emotional complaints. What is consistently found is that psychotherapy is generally effective; that the most important factors are those inherent to the patient involving his or her resources and the quality of the relationship between patient and therapist as rated by the patient.[35] Current approaches in most psychiatric services, including Child and Adolescent Mental Health Services (CAMHS), haven't yet caught up with what the research findings are saying and tend to emphasise process 'standardisation' through following 'how to do it' technical approaches to psychiatric problems, with diagnostic-specific treatment approaches. However, specific technique is a factor shown to have as much as seven times less influence on outcome than the 'common' (to all psychotherapeutic approaches) factor of the quality of the therapeutic alliance as rated by the client.

What this means for a service user is that it is much more important that you strike up a good relationship with a clinician whose approach 'makes sense' to you than getting a diagnosis and receiving a specific therapy tailored to that diagnosis. It could be that you prefer and would feel more comfortable with a therapist of a particular gender or ethnic background, or that you prefer to talk about what's going on emotionally, or that you want someone who gives you tasks to do and is very practical, or perhaps someone who would see all the family to facilitate communication etc. We each have ideas about what it is we might need to improve our situation or help us solve a difficult problem. Good therapy is about being able to match up our beliefs with a therapist who you feel 'knows where you're coming from'. That's what the evidence says and that's what many years of clinical experience confirms for me.

To help you decide on what sort of approach you might find makes sense for you, below I've listed some common therapeutic approaches you may come across in a typical Child and Adolescent Mental Health Service (CAMHS):

Family therapy – Usually involves meeting with various family members in various combinations to explore family relationships, understand the dynamics of these relationships and make suggestions on how to change these dynamics for the better.

Systemic therapy – Is an extension of family therapy as it involves working with other significant people beyond the family, for example, schools, friends, extended family, employers, social services, other professionals and so on.

Behaviour therapy – Commonly used for behaviour problems and usually involves working with parents to develop strategies based on analysing the problem behaviours and then devising various consequences (rewards and punishments) to reduce unwanted behaviours and increase the desired ones.

Cognitive therapy – Based on looking at a person's thoughts to help them analyse how their thought processes may be causing emotional and behavioural problems and from this analysis to help them change their thought processes in a more positive direction. Very often cognitive therapy methods are used in combination with behaviour therapy methods, and the term cognitive behaviour therapy (CBT) is widely used to describe this combintion of approaches.

Psychodynamic psychotherapy – Based on understanding how emotional conflicts arise including from traumatic experiences and thus helping the person process unresolved emotional issues.

Group therapy – Involves a variety of techniques including all the above, but using a format of having people together in a group where they have an opportunity to learn from each other and provide support for each other.

It is worth mentioning that these approaches are not mutually exclusive and usually involve a lot of crossover, for example, a cognitive therapist doesn't usually ignore emotional conflicts, nor does a psychodynamic therapist usually ignore thought processes. The differences are often ones of emphasis and in real-life clinical encounters many therapists (often without realising it) 'mix and match' bringing in aspects of different models to fit whatever the persons or persons they are working with brings.

Other approaches

There are a whole variety of other approaches including those focusing on diet and nutrition, exercise, lifestyle and so on (I mention a few in the next chapter). Most competent doctors and therapists will be able to combine a range of therapuetic approaches in a way that combines with and makes sense to the patient.

Summary

In this chapter I introduced the reader to common treatments used for childhood psychiatric disorders. I presented the evidence that shows that the three main classes of drugs used – antidepressants, stimulants, and antipsychotics – are not particularly effective (in the long term) nor safe and therefore should not, in my opinion, be used as a first-line treatment or by doctors not familiar with the scientific literature.

Psychotherapy in contrast is effective and safe, however, there is little evidence to support the idea that particular psychotherapy techniques make a big difference to achieving a positive outcome and much evidence to suggest that the quality of the relationship between therapist/doctor and patient does.

Chapter 5
Summary and getting help

In the series introduction (pp. v–x), the aims, scope and style of the approach taken are introduced. Let me summarise the main arguments in the subsequent chapters of this book:

• In Chapter 1 I argued that our understanding of childhood distress and children's mental health (including the scientific investigation of this) is shaped by the cultural beliefs of a society. These cultural beliefs are influenced by our value systems and these in turn influence the meaning we give to a problem and what we then do about it. I introduced the term 'social construction' to describe this process and explained how our beliefs about what constitutes a 'normal' and 'abnormal' childhood (and child rearing) are socially constructed.

• In Chapter 2 I presented some figures illustrating that there has been a rapid increase in the amount of psychiatric drugs being prescribed to the young. I suggested that this could be interpreted as a symptom of a 'dysfunctional' culture rather than due to scientific progress uncovering previously unrecognised disorders and treating them. I discussed a number of recent cultural changes that have affected children and explored the impact that a narcissistic value system has on children and families. I briefly explored globalisation seeing in it threats and new risks for children and families but also new opportunities for positive learning.

• In Chapter 3 I argued that childhood psychiatric diagnoses have little scientific evidence to support the idea that they represent physical disorders of the brain and nervous system. Using three increasingly common diagnoses (ADHD, autism, and childhood depression) as examples I analysed some of the 'scientific' evidence from a critical point of view to conclude that these diagnoses (like other childhood psychiatric diagnoses but unlike proven physical conditions) tell you very little (possibly nothing) about the cause, treatment, and outcome for an emotional or behavioural problem.

• In Chapter 4 I introduced the reader to common treatments used for childhood psychiatric disorders. I presented the evidence that shows that the three main classes of drugs used – antidepressants, stimulants, and antipsychotics – are neither effective (in the long term) nor safe, and should therefore not, in my opinion, be used as a first-line treatment or by doctors not familiar with this literature. Psychotherapy in contrast is effective and safe, however, there is little evidence to support the idea that particular psychotherapy techniques make a big difference to achieving a positive outcome and much evidence to suggest that the quality of the relationship between therapist/doctor and patient does.

So what does this all mean for you, if you are reading this to try and understand a problem you or your child is struggling with? Before discussing potential professional help and what to look for in this, here are a few things that may be helpful to consider first, to help you solve whatever problem you are facing.

Common pitfalls

After reading about the social construction of childhood and how our expectations of children have increased and our ideas about what makes a 'normal' child narrowed, you may have already decided that you wish to worry less about your child and focus more on the positives. If, however, you have got to this point, remain concerned, and are looking for ways to make progress with your child, then have a look through the list below of 'common pitfalls' that can 'interfere' with whatever approach you are taking to try and solve a problem.

Giving up too quickly

It is important that you make a commitment to see through whatever intervention or strategy you have decided to try and not give up on the strategy if you feel that you are not getting anywhere after a few days. This is particularly so for food supplements where you may have to wait for as long as two or three months whilst the supplement is working, repairing and improving the functioning of cells, before changes are observed. With some of the interventions like behavioural interventions, the use of negative consequences (punishments) for unwanted behaviour often means that unwanted behaviours actually get worse before they start to improve. This is because if you are putting boundaries around negative behaviour and the child does not like this, then they may feel they have to go even further than usual in their negative behaviour in order to get you to give in. However, keep in mind that the vast majority of children will feel happier and safer once any system that you are using has had time to 'bed in' and they have got used to the new rules boundaries and are regularly getting positive consequences for good behaviour.

Becoming hopeless following a setback

Setbacks are an inevitable part of any recovery process. There are many reasons why people experience setbacks. This can include the normal ups and downs of life, 'taking your eye off the ball' resulting in a slackening off of the strategies that you were using, and upsetting experiences that cause deterioration in mood and/or behaviour. Whatever the reason, setbacks are so common that they inevitably occur at some point. What often happens when a setback occurs is that parents, the child, the teacher (or whoever it is affecting) feel demoralised, and think something like 'what was the point of all of the things that we just did as we are back at square one now'. At this point, hopelessness creeps in and with it a sense of failure and a loss of confidence in the ability to bring about lasting change. When the inevitable setback occurs therefore, it is important to remember that your reaction of demoralisation and despair are perfectly normal, that what is happening is what usually happens and that, far from being back at square one, whatever improvement had occurred is a fact that cannot be taken away. If there has been a period of improved mood or behaviour then this means you have already learnt new skills. These skills will help you deal with new situations and setbacks as they arrive. When the inevitable setback occurs have a think about what might be happening, talk to someone close about it, and return to those strategies that have been successful in the past, or adjust them to suit the new circumstances better.

Unrealistic expectations

If we have unrealistic expectations of our children's behaviour, then we will continue to feel disappointed with them. Your disappointment may be felt by your child through the various ways your frustration and disappointment are shown. This can include negative comments towards your child about them. In addition, the emotional upset your disappointment may cause is often noticed by children. A difficult question to answer is 'how do I know if my expectations are unreasonable?' Of course, this is never going to be a straightforward question with a straightforward answer, and will vary from individual to individual. Our relationships are always multi-dimensional and there are always likely to be bits of our expectations (in any relationship, not just with our children) that are a mixture of reasonable and unreasonable. In helping you try and 'unpack' whether there are particular areas of unreasonable expectation that may be hindering your relationship with your children, here are a few things to consider:

- Are you expecting your child to stop expressing their emotions? The emotion we find hardest as parents is that of anger. Anger, however, is a strong and, indeed, energising emotion. It can be unhealthy to suppress it. It is usually better to try and help our children find ways to express anger that are not going to harm people around them. This is hard for any adult to do, let only children (I'm sure a moment's self-reflection will confirm this!). Therefore, whilst becoming calm, having total control over anger, and not getting angry is an unreasonable expectation, encouraging your child to express anger (and other emotions) in ways that are non-harmful to others is a reasonable expectation. Note how well you yourself are able to control anger and whether at times you are expecting your child to do something you find difficult. This can be a good guide as to whether your expectations are unreasonable.

- Are you expecting to get rid of negative emotion? Whilst it is a reasonable expectation and, indeed I would argue, a vital necessity, to have a relationship with your child which is underpinned by positive emotion and love towards them, it is unreasonable to expect an absence of negative feelings, such as anger, hostility and, indeed, shame in that relationship. A mixture of positive and negative feelings is present in any meaningful relationship and the presence of negative feelings does not mean your relationship is in trouble. It is very common for children when they are angry and upset with you to say 'nasty' things about you or themselves such as 'you are the worst mummy/daddy in the world' or 'I wish I was never born'. Try not to take these negative expressions too personally, or as being part of a permanent feeling.

• Can you separate behaviour which is the result of poor comprehension or misunderstanding from that which is simply due to disobedience? Questions to ask here are: does your child have a particular learning disability, or has your child not been listening to your instructions (for example, have you been getting them to repeat what you say to make sure that they have understood what you are asking)? If your child does not understand your instructions, then they cannot follow through what you are asking of them. Over long periods this may become a source of frustration and unfulfilled expectations.

• Are you expecting a boy to stop being boisterous? Boys and girls are different. Fathers may find it hard to relate to girl's behaviour and mothers may find it hard to relate to typical boy behaviour. Boys are naturally more impulsive, physically active, and aggressive than girls. Of course, this does not mean that all boys are like this or that all girls aren't. However, if you are trying to eliminate the impulsiveness, levels of activity and aggression of some children who are naturally more boisterous, then you will be likely to feel disappointed.

Inconsistency

Most parents know about this but it is worth restating. Children are often clever enough to spot opportunities to further their own desires. If mum tells their child they are not allowed to, let's say, go out and visit their friend because they have misbehaved, then it is a common strategy for them to go to the other parent and ask them if they can go and see their friend, particularly if they know that their dad is more likely to say yes. Therefore, before trying to apply any strategy, talk to your partner or any other person who is important and involved in the care of your child to discuss what approach you're taking. Discuss any strategies you are thinking of implementing with them to make sure that you are in agreement and that you will support each other and back each other up as you work through your problems. Of course 100% consistency is very rare and a degree of inconsistency is part of life; indeed, it would be very boring if all our relationships existed with people who were just like us (as much as sometimes we wish this in fantasy)! This brings me to my next common pitfall.

Unresolved difficulties between parents

If there are unresolved difficulties of a serious nature between parents and/or carers of the child (whether they are together or separated) then these will often show themselves through the emotional state and behaviour of their children. This is where issues such as inconsistency can become a potentially serious obstacle to progress. Furthermore, it is not just serious, unresolved difficulties between parents, but also between you and others involved extensively in the care of that child; for example, an unresolved difficulty between a parent and a grandparent who also does a lot of caring for the child. Although it is beyond the scope of this book to deal with all the different types of problems that carers may have in their relationships with each other, the key to establishing working solutions to these types of problems is for decisions to rest with the immediate parents or carers of the child, coupled with communication and compromise.

In a situation where the parental couple have separated, it is vital to put any continuing animosity towards one another to one side, to keep the child out of any arguments, and not use the child in any way as a tool to express hostility towards an ex-partner. Sometimes when there are disputes in the parental relationship, parents may recruit one of their children as an ally against the other parent. This can happen whether the parents are still together or separated. In this situation the parent will say negative things about the other parent to their child, which can result in split loyalties for the child. In this situation you should try to arrive at business-like agreements on what common strategies to use and what ways of communicating with each other about the child that there will be. This may require a third party (an outsider to the relationship) to help you negotiate this, whether this be a professional or a trusted acquaintance.

I have sometimes heard it said in my clinical sessions that it is the child's behaviour that has caused the marriage to split or caused problems in the parent's relationship. Whilst I accept that some behaviour problems make parents feel ill, I think that such a conclusion should be avoided. As parents we have, and should have, a more powerful position in the relationship with our children. In typical family systems, the parents should be in charge – they have to be the boss. With this power comes responsibility. In the same way that we, as parents, are trying to teach our children to take responsibility for their behaviour, we too as adults have to take responsibility for our actions and decisions. Not only is it unreasonable to pass the burden on to our children through blaming them for causing any difficulties we are experiencing in our parental relationships, but also expecting to solve our parental relationships by getting rid of behaviours which we don't want to see in our children sets everyone up for failure. It's also worth keeping in mind that sometimes children misbehave or develop an emotional problem as a (unconscious) way of keeping parents together when there is a fear that the parents may separate (as parents then focus their attention on the problems that the child is having rather than on the problems between themselves).

Unresolved issues from your own childhood

All parents were children once and many of the parents I see in my clinical practice had difficult childhoods or are carrying issues from their past that, for whatever reason, remain unresolved. By itself this is not a reason why any particular approach or strategy would not work; however, it is worth reflecting on this, as it may help you identify emotional obstacles that prevent you from carrying out strategies that may prove to be effective. For example, if you had a poor relationship with your own parents that led you to hate or fear them, you may, once you became a parent yourself, have decided that you were going to make sure your children don't grow up to have the same poor image of you that you had of your parents – in other words, that they don't grow up to hate or fear you. This may, without you necessarily realising it, have led you to avoid 'upsetting' your children, because of a fear that this will lead them to hate you (which is the thing you're trying to avoid). In turn, this means that you might get stuck when it comes to some strategies that involve being able to tolerate upsetting your children and them saying horrible things like they 'hate you' (for example, when using negative consequences [punishments] for unacceptable behaviour). Search within yourself to try and identify whether your own childhood experiences may make some things difficult because of the emotions they provoke.

The scapegoat child

I often liken families to a drama or play. In most families we find that, over time, people establish their role and position in that family. It is as if we each have a script and for the family system to function everybody has a different script and always uses their own particular script or role in that play. Upset is created in a family if somebody steps out of their usual script as everyone else then becomes unsure of what their lines are. This seems to be true whether a family has got a good, well-functioning script or a terrible and problematic one. This is where the phenomena of 'scapegoating' can happen without anyone being aware that it's going on. There is a humorous example of this in a series of children's books that my children have enjoyed for some years. The books are about a boy called *Horrid Henry*, who is always badly behaved. *Horrid Henry* has a brother who is called *Perfect Peter* because he is, in contrast to *Horrid Henry*, always so well behaved. The script in this particular family is that *Horrid Henry* is always naughty and gets told off and *Perfect Peter* is always, in contrast to this, good and used to being told good things about his behaviour. Generally, of course, both children live up to these expectations. In this particular story *Horrid Henry* decided not to follow his usual 'script' and to try his best to be good for the day. As the day goes on *Perfect Peter* finds it harder and harder to cope with the fact that *Horrid Henry* is not being told off. *Perfect Peter* finds this change of script very difficult. *Perfect Peter* tries to keep provoking *Horrid Henry* into being 'nasty' towards him (an attempt if you like to return this family to its usual 'script'). *Horrid Henry* refuses to rise to the bait as he is being good that day and eventually *Perfect Peter* is so frustrated by this he ends up doing something very obviously naughty so that he ends up being told off and *Horrid Henry* praised.

This story is certainly familiar for many families where there tends to be one sibling who is the 'naughty' one. However, if it becomes another sibling's turn to be the naughty one, then the sibling who is usually naughty often becomes good. So it is useful to ask yourself whether the child you are most concerned about is playing the part of the 'naughty' or 'depressed' or 'anxious' (etc.) child in the family system and this has become his or her script. As you might find in many school playgrounds, other siblings may use various strategies (such as winding them up, or always telling on them, trying to protect them and so on) to keep them in that familiar role. If you think this may be the case then keep a keen eye out for how other siblings/family members/friends may be provoking the one you are most concerned about to stay in their role.

The anger–guilt–reparation cycle

See if you recognise this pattern. You are infuriated with your child's behaviour and in your anger you scold him or her and impose some sort of punishment (anger). Later you calm down and feel guilty for what you have done and so feel you have acted unfairly and that your punishments where unduly harsh (guilt). As a result you try to repair some of the damage that you feel you have done in your anger and therefore give the child that you have felt you have treated badly some sort of treat or comfort, essentially to make yourself feel better (reparation). It is worth noting here that this cycle can also occur in children too, who may similarly go through an anger–guilt–reparation cycle. Whilst, in itself, this is a perfectly normal and, in some ways, a healthy thing to be able to do, it can become a problem when this becomes the usual pattern with which conflicts with your child are dealt with and the way in which consequences are imposed. The child learns that any consequences imposed may be withdrawn and, indeed, may be followed by some sort of reward. Thus, commonly, behaviour deteriorates after the special treat or period of comforting, you feel furious with the child again for not responding positively to your 'treat' or attempt to comfort them and you go back into the anger–guilt–reparation cycle.

If you recognise this cycle, then try and have, ready to hand, simple consequences that you know you will be able to stick to, and if you feel that your behaviour towards your child when you were angry was unacceptable, then the healthy way to do the 'reparation' is to make a sincere apology to your child, explaining carefully what aspects of your behaviour towards the child you felt were unacceptable, but not minimising whatever behaviour you felt was unacceptable from your child. By doing this, you are also modelling the ability to take responsibility for your own behaviour.

Not using the strategies for all of your children

Whilst some strategies may be specific to one of your children with whom you are having difficulties (for example, some dietary interventions), others should be used for all of your children (such as consequences for good or bad behaviour), as otherwise you risk the child with the problems feeling that they are being unfairly picked on.

Hostility towards your child

In some situations the predominant feeling towards your child may have become that of hostility, rejection and anger (in other words a predominantly negative and rejecting emotion towards your child). There are many reasons why this may have become so. Maybe you had an unhappy childhood and the behaviours of your child remind you of painful, unhappy things in your own childhood – things that you are trying to forget. It could be that your child's behaviour reminds of you of an unhappy and painful relationship in your adult life, for example, a child reminds you of his or her father who was aggressive and bullying towards you. Or it may be that years of difficulty with your child's behaviour have 'soured' your relationship with your child.

Whatever the reason, if there is a predominantly negative and hostile set of feelings towards your child, it is highly likely that your child will know this and feel insecure in their relationship with you. This can have many consequences. The child can come to view themselves as bad, unlovable, or unlikable. At the same time, because you have mainly negative feelings towards this child, it will become increasingly difficult to notice positive aspects of your child and so your attention will be routinely drawn to those things that confirm your negative view of your child. This can quickly become a mutually reinforcing, negative cycle – in other words, your child feels rejected and becomes angry and rejecting, thus confirming your negative impression of your child, leading to you having hostile and rejecting feelings towards them, and so on. If you recognise this situation then pay particular attention to finding opportunities to build a more positive and a more loving relationship with your child, making a special effort to start noticing the positives.

Inadvertently supporting the creation of a 'safe zone'

We are exposed to constant messages telling us how dangerous the outside world is, particularly for children. It is a very normal response to then try to protect our children as much as we can from exposure to unpleasant and traumatic experiences such as bullying and drug abuse. The result has been something that some call 'the domestication of children', where it has been observed that children are increasingly confined to the home environment or indoor settings at school where their behaviour and actions can be monitored much more closely. This desire to wrap our children in 'cotton wool' and protect them from the dangers of the world 'out there', is completely understandable, but not necessarily very helpful in allowing children to develop the resilience that they may need to cope with the reality of the world they find themselves in. Learn to let your children go, and cope with the anxiety it causes you.

Fear of change

As I mentioned above under 'scapegoating', families have a tendency towards repeating a particular script, where everybody has their own role (whether people like their role or not). When somebody starts changing their role it challenges the whole family script, leaving other individuals in the family feeling uncertain about how the new script works. In these circumstances there is a natural tendency to want to return back to the familiar script (even unhappy ones – it is a kind of 'better the devil you know than the devil you don't'). It is a familiar experience for many of us in clinical practice that with some families, the advice given is not acted upon by them – or only half-heartedly. There are many reasons for this including some of the ones outlined above. However, one important reason worth thinking about is whether you fear change. This can be change in how you think, what you do, how you manage time in your family's lifestyles, in personal ambitions and so on. Change always includes a certain amount of anxiety and fear of the unknown, not just for the individual but also the other family members, as the usual 'family script' is disturbed. Be aware of this and embrace the excitement that can accompany reaching into the unknown and the new possibilities for your life that may be opened up by this.

Lack of support

As the old African saying reminds us 'it takes a village to raise a child'. Life as a parent seems harder than ever these days; not only are there higher expectations with regards our children's behaviour and a close watch kept on our behaviour as parents by various agencies of the state, but also our family and community support networks have dwindled. Raising children demands a lot from us, both physically and mentally, and given the pressures on us to behave in particular ways as parents, more than ever we now need trusted partners, friends and other family members to provide us with both emotional and practical support to share the burden of responsibility.

Lack of time

Another feature of modern life is how busy and time stretched we are. Working hours have increased over the past few decades and it is the norm now in two-parent households for both parents to work. When we are not working we are often busy trying to complete the necessary household chores, like cleaning and shopping, leaving less and less time for us to spend with our children and to give them the sort of attention they crave. With trying to complete so many things with such little time we have more and more reasons to feel stressed.

This pattern may have been less of a problem in times gone by and in other cultures, where children grew up surrounded by other children. Having regular, easily available playmates (as I did as a child growing up in Iraq) means that there is less need for the adults to be available as the providers of fun time. Sadly, the way our culture in the West has developed means that a decrease in the amount of time parents are spending in their families is coinciding with the increasing domestication of children (in other words children increasingly being confined to places where there is constant adult supervision, such as schools, clubs and home, due to the fears I mentioned above). Try looking at your usual routines, work hours and so on to see if you can make more time to spend with your family if this is lacking.

Unresolved trauma

Of course, everybody reacts differently to trauma (be this abuse, loss of a parent, being assaulted, involved in a serious accident, etc.) and each particular person's circumstances have different features. For some, trauma may lead them to feel preoccupied, constantly worrying about their safety and the safety of others and therefore they will present with poor concentration and matters such as school work will be of limited importance to them. Others may have developed the psychological defence of 'being on the go', that is by constantly doing things it keeps their minds away from thinking and worrying about what has happened and what may happen to them in the future. Others still may find the school a sanctuary, away from whatever unhappy situation they are experiencing, and their difficulties only become obvious in the home setting.

The most important factor to help children who have experienced trauma is having a secure, stable and loving social environment. It is not, contrary to what some may believe, the provision of special therapy for a child who has been traumatised (though this is certainly helpful for some children).

Coming off medication

Some of you reading this book will have a child who is taking psychiatric medication. Having read this book, some of you may decide that you wish to take your child off this medication. Although it's advisable to consult a doctor before coming off medication, the decision on whether to withdraw your child's medication rests with you. Many people find that their doctor won't agree with your decision. A study for the UK national mental health charity 'Mind' (the study was with adults who wished to discontinue their psychiatric medications) found that, in practice, doctors were often unhelpful. Many thus decided to come off medication against the advice of their doctors, or without involving them in the decision. Furthermore, when coming off their medications, the most helpful people were those who had no role in prescribing their medication, such as other service users, self-help groups, and complementary therapists. Doctors seemed to be less concerned than service users about the side effects of medication, less understanding of their desire to live without drugs, and more likely to doubt their ability to do so successfully.[1] So if you have taken the decision to take your child off medication, don't let the disagreement of your doctor necessarily put you off.

When weaning a child off any psychiatric medication, you should bear in mind that some withdrawal symptoms are likely. This is because psychiatric medicines act at the nerve endings of brain cells, and the result of their action is to increase or decrease the amount of a certain chemical involved in relaying signals from one brain cell to another (a neurotransmitter). What often then happens after a while of this change in the amount of neurotransmitter is that brain cells start changing to adjust to the new levels of neurotransmitter. For example, if a drug has caused an increase in neurotransmitter levels, then, over time, the brain cell receiving this neurotransmitter will start reducing the number of receptors (that receive the signal from this neurotransmitter) that it has in reaction to the increase in this chemical. This is why for many people the psychological effects of psychiatric drugs tend to wear off over time, often leading to gradually increasing doses being given. It also means that withdrawing the drug suddenly is not recommended.

The general 'rule of thumb' is that if your child has been taking a psychiatric drug for over three months then wean them off gradually over a period of eight to ten weeks. Below three months this can be done quicker. If your child is taking a long-acting preparation (such as the stimulant Concerta), then ask your doctor to switch your child to the equivalent dose of a short-acting preparation (in Concerta's case this will be Ritalin or Equasym), which will then be easier to adjust.

For example, let's suppose your child is taking 40mg a day of Ritalin. A 'weaning off' regime may then look like this (it will involve using a sharp knife to cut the 10mg tablets):

- *Week 1:* Go to 35mg per day in divided doses, starting with reducing the last dose of the day. Dividing the doses depends on what your current regime is. If, for example, the regime is 20mg first thing in the morning and 20mg at lunch time, then the first step will be 20mg in the morning as before, but reduce the lunch time dose to 15mg. If your regime is a three-times-a-day one, for example, 15mg in the morning 15mg at lunch and 10mg late afternoon, then cut the late afternoon dose to 5mg.

- *Week 2:* Now go to 30mg per day in divided doses. In this example it would mean 15mg twice a day if you are on the twice-a-day regime, or 15, 10 and 5mg if you are on the three-times-a-day regime.

- *Week 3:* Now go to 25mg per day in divided doses. This would mean 15mg in the morning 10mg at lunch time on the twice-a-day regime and 10, 10, and 5mg on the three-times-a-day regime example.

- *Week 4:* Now go to 20mg per day in divided doses. 10 and 10mg for twice a day; 10, 5 and 5mg for three times a day.

- *Weeks 5 and 6:* Now go to 15mg per day in divided doses. 10 and 5mg for twice a day; 5, 5 and 5mg for three times a day.

- *Weeks 7 and 8:* Now go to 10mg per day in divided doses. 5 and 5mg for twice a day; and 5 and 5mg for three times a day, cutting out the late afternoon dose.

- *Weeks 9 and 10:* Now go to 5mg per day (morning only).

- *Week 11:* Discontinue.

If your child is taking more than one medication, then work out a weaning-off regime for each one, and then do the withdrawal programme for each, one by one, rather than at the same time. If one drug has been prescribed for the side effects of another, then start with the original drug. For example, if an antidepressant has been prescribed after a stimulant (which may have caused the low mood), start by first withdrawing the original drug, in this case the stimulant, and then the subsequent drug, in this case the antidepressant. Some drugs (like some antidepressants) come in capsule form which cannot be divided into smaller amounts. In this case use a reducing regime that includes having the capsule every other day (once you are down to one capsule a day) and then one every third day.

Five simple things to try

1. Diet and nutrition: As the old saying reminds us 'healthy in body, healthy in mind'. Modern children's diets are high in sugars, fats, and salt and low in fibre, vitamins and minerals, and essential fatty acids. There are three components to improving young peoples' nutrition that have evidence to support them improving their mental health. Firstly, eliminate potential irritants – try removing all artificial additives and where possible use organic or free-range foods and home cooking rather than pre-prepared meals and fast foods. Secondly, add any missing nutrients – try a daily multivitamin and mineral supplement and daily supplement of essential fatty acids (particularly the Omega 3 'EPA' and evening primrose oil) such as Eye-Q or Vegepa. Thirdly, balance the diet – reduce sugars and saturated fats (unless the person is suffering from anorexia and so needs the calories), increase complex carbohydrates (which help regulate blood sugar levels) and fibre (through raw fruit and vegetables) and have three balanced meals a day (don't miss breakfast).

2. Fresh air and exercise: Enable your child(ren) to get plenty of opportunities for exercise (particularly outdoors) including chances for unstructured and unsupervised active play.

3. Clear and consistent consequences: Two catch phrases are worth remembering 'Catch your child being good' and 'Stay firm, keep calm'. Use positive consequences for good behaviour and work hard to find opportunities to praise, notice or reward your child when they are good (Catch your child being good). Notice your child's strengths and support and encourage these in a positive direction. Use negative consequences for unwanted behaviour and work hard to stick to these and not give in (Stay firm, keep calm). When giving these negative consequences (such as time out, and withdrawal of privileges) make sure that you are threatening the child with things you know you can stick to and are fairly immediate. Make sure you are being reasonable, are in control of what you are doing, and be aware of what the laws of your country say you can or cannot do (for example some countries have outlawed the use of physical punishments). Try not to get drawn into arguments, which often just feed further emotional energy and attention, making the situation worse.

4. Regular positive family time: Find opportunities to do things together as a family on a regular basis, for example going out together once every weekend and having at least one meal together a day. Like all relationships we have to continue 'working' on our relationships with our children – year after year after year after …

5. Communication and understanding: Talk to each other, but more importantly *listen* to each other (not the same thing). Try and understand your child's point of view and help them understand yours. Try and create regular opportunities for you to communicate, listen and try and understand what's on each of your minds.

Remember the above are just ideas and suggestions. Some of them may make sense and so work for you; others may not and may not be relevant to your situation. There isn't one magic 'cure-all' that works for everyone. Furthermore, as I am both writing for a predominantly Western and British audience and this is also the culture in which I live and was trained, the suggestions are bound to have a bias toward the attitudes, beliefs and practices of modern British-Western culture, and some ideas may not necessarily translate well into other cultures or settings.

Some of you may have already got to the point or will get to the point of needing to seek further help. This is OK. It is an important skill for us to know when we need the help of others and accept this. Accepting the need for help is often a sign of greater courage and honesty than avoiding it.

Finding the right professional

As I mentioned in the last chapter, the good news is that psychotherapeutic approaches are effective and can make an important and positive difference to peoples' lives. Many of those in the 'helping' professions have been drawn to the profession because of a wish to help those who are experiencing suffering and so the vast majority are caring, thoughtful, and trustworthy people. Of course there are problems, as with any profession, of some 'rogue' elements, and child psychiatry has been somewhat tainted as I described earlier by the lure of money from the drug companies. However, I believe the majority are decent, hardworking people who genuinely care and are doing their best to try and help those they see (and this includes those who disagree with the opinions expressed in this book).

The starting point for most people in the UK who are experiencing mental health problems is the family doctor (General Practitioner – GP). If you are experiencing emotional or behavioural problems with your child then they are likely to refer you to Child and Adolescent Mental Health Services (CAMHS) or a community paediatrician. Some GP practices have counsellors in their practice, some of whom may also see children and families. Others pathways to professional help for emotional and behavioural problems in the young include schools, social services, the voluntary sector, and private therapists.

Child and Adolescent Mental Health Services (CAMHS) – Sometimes called Child and Family Services (CAFS)
CAMHS services are multidisciplinary services (having a range of different disciplines working in them) that have 'specialists' with training in child and adolescent mental health problems. Different teams have different professionals. Who is in any particular team largely depends on local circumstances (such as funding levels, ease of recruitment, availability of any particular professional group, any training or research activities going on there and so on). Different professionals working in CAMHS teams include:

- *Child and adolescent psychiatrists:* psychiatrists first qualify as doctors (and therefore have knowledge about physical disorders, can order physical investigations such as blood tests, and can prescribe medication) before going on to train as psychiatrists and then child and adolescent psychiatrists.

- *Clinical psychologists:* have taken a first degree in psychology (the scientific study of human behaviour and the mind) and then trained in clinical psychology (psychology as applied to clinical situations).

- *Psychotherapists:* have completed training in a model of psychotherapy. Psychiatrists, psychologists, social workers, specialist nurses, etc., may also be psychotherapists, but psychotherapists are not necessarily any of those professions originally.

- *Social workers:* have trained to become a social worker and then completed specialist training or gained adequate experience in child and adolescent mental health.

- *Specialist nurses:* have completed the training to become a 'registered mental nurse' and then completed specialist training or gained adequate experience in child and adolescent mental health.

- *Others:* A variety of other professionals may be found in different CAMHS teams including family therapists (some CAMHS teams have family therapy as a separate sub-speciality and not under 'psychotherapy'), art therapists, occupational therapists, educational psychologists (who, unlike clinical psychologists, usually focus on educational rather than emotional difficulties), and specialist teachers.

CAMHS services also run adolescent inpatient units which are residential assessment and treatment facilities for cases of a more serious nature, such as those with a psychosis (where young people may be hearing voices, experiencing delusions, intense paranoia or their thinking has become seriously distorted or bizarre), are suicidal, or have a serious eating disorder or who have become stuck and are not making progress despite extensive input.

Paediatrics

Many community (as opposed to hospital) paediatricians run clinics for behavioural disorders where conditions such as ADHD and autism will be diagnosed. Referral can come directly from the GP but also occurs through 'medical officers' who are doctors attached to schools. As I have explained earlier, in my opinion, paediatricians on the whole do not have the right background training, qualifications or knowledge (for example, of the literature I have reviewed in this book) to assess, understand and intervene psychotherapeutically with behavioural problems. Usually assessments are confined to questions of diagnosis, and treatments tend to revolve around the use of medication. My recommendation therefore is that on the whole (of course there is variability in personality, approach, etc. as in any professional group), you are better off getting a referral to a CAMHS team than paediatrics for any emotional or/and behavioural problem with your child.

School
If the problem is solely or primarily school based, then it is preferable to get the school or education authority to help you resolve this. Schools have several services that they can call on to help them with a particular pupil or problem. These include the Emotional Behavioural Support Service (EBSS) who help the school devise strategies for pupils with emotional and/or behavioural problems, and educational psychologists who can assess pupils for learning difficulties or other behavioural and academic issues. Some schools also employ school counsellors. In addition, all schools and education authorities should have policies and procedures for issues such as bullying. Children in the UK with persistent issues relating to either their learning or their behaviour should be given an 'Individual Education Plan' (IEP), which, if the difficulties are severe enough, can lead to an application for a 'Statement' of special educational needs. A statement provides pupils with extra input such as extra teaching, support, mentoring, or even attendance at a specialised school.

Social services
Anyone can request input from social services, but their involvement tends to be about issues such as child protection (where there is a concern about the safety of a child and whether they are being subjected to 'abuse' [the four categories

of child abuse are: sexual abuse, physical abuse, emotional abuse, and neglect, although the definition for each is often open to interpretation]), family support (particularly for families with a disabled child), fostering and adoption, and parenting support and advice.

Voluntary

The voluntary sector includes a variety of organisations that vary from locality to locality. Some may have been set up to support the needs of particular groups (e.g., particular ethnic minority communities) others may be national (such as Young Minds, Parentline, and the National Autistic Society). Find out about what's available in your locality through the local council, library or social services.

Finally there is a whole variety of *private therapists* who may be qualified and/or experienced in working with children and families. Whichever path you take, remember that if you are receiving therapy for an emotional and/or behavioural problem with your child, then striking up a positive and trusting relationship is strongly linked in the evidence to a subsequent positive outcome. However, there is one proviso worth remembering about this. You can have a situation where you have a very good relationship with your doctor/therapist but matters don't improve. This is rarer than a poor relationship leading then to a poor outcome, but it is just as problematic. In either case, if matters are not improving it is your right to ask for a change of therapist, and good therapists accept that not everyone will be a 'good fit' with them. Try and avoid working simultaneously with two different people (unless they are from the same team and clearly work closely together) as this can cause unnecessary confusion and potential contradictions that are often counter-productive.

Summary

In this, the final chapter of this book, I have focused more on the practical things families with young people in distress can do. This has included presenting issues to think about and five simple things to try before seeking professional help. Finally I provided a brief summary of different professional services and groups available from a UK-based perspective.

Endnotes

Chapter 1

1. Page 10 in Clarke, J, Hall, S, Jefferson, T & Roberts, B (1975) Subcultures, cultures and class. In S Hall & T Jefferson (Eds) *Resistance through Rituals: Youth subcultures in post-war Britain.* London: Hutchinson.

2. See for example Hartmann, T (2008) Good science, expectations, villains and hope. In S Timimi & J Leo (Eds) *Rethinking ADHD* (pp 398–412). Basingstoke: Palgrave MacMillan; and Barkley, R (2000) More on evolution, hunting, and ADHD. *The ADHD Report, 8*, 2, 1–7.

3. See Thom Hartmann's website <http://www.thomhartmann.com>. Accessed 03.03.2008.

4. See <http://www.adhdrelief.com/famous.html>. Accessed 03.03.2008.

5. Timimi, S (2005) *Naughty Boys: Anti-social behaviour, ADHD, and the role of culture.* Basingstoke: Palgrave MacMillan.

6. Aries, P (1962) *Centuries of Childhood.* London: Jonathan Cape.

7. Elias, N (1939/1978) *The Civilizing Process.* New York: Blackwell.

8. Erasmus, D (1985) *The Collected Works of Erasmus, Vol 25.* Toronto: University of Toronto Press.

9. You can find more detail and full references in my 2005 book: *Naughty Boys: Anti-social behaviour, ADHD and the role of culture.* Basingstoke: Palgrave MacMillan.

Chapter 2

1. Wong, IC, Murray, ML, Camilleri-Novak, D & Stephens, P (2004) Increased prescribing trends of paediatric psychotropic medications. *Archives of Disease in Childhood, 89*, 1131–2.

2. Olfson, M, Marcus, SC, Weissman, MM & Jensen, PS (2002) National trends in the use of psychotropic medications by children. *Journal of the American Academy of Child and Adolescent Psychiatry, 41*, 514–21; and Zito, JM, Safer, DJ, Dosreis, S, Gardner, JF, Boles, J & Lynch, F (2000) Trends in prescribing of psychotropic medication in pre-schoolers. *Journal of the American Medical Association, 283*, 1025–30.

3. This can be found from UK Department of Health figures at: Prescription Cost Analysis England 2004. Department of Health, NHSE, 2005. Available at <http://www.dh.gov.uk/PublicationsAndStatistics/Publications/ PublicationsStatistics/PublicationsStatisticsArticle/fs en?CONTENT_ID=4107504&chk=nsvFE0>. Accessed 03.03.2008.

4. See <http://www.usatoday.com/news/health/2006-05-01-atypical-drugs_x.htm>. Accessed 03.03.2008.

5. See for example the following report: British Medical Association (2006) *Child and Adolescent Mental Health: A guide for professionals*. London: BMA.

6. You can find more detail and full references in my 2005 book: *Naughty Boys: Anti-social behaviour, ADHD and the role of culture*. Basingstoke: Palgrave MacMillan.

7. Wolfenstein, M (1955) Fun morality: An analysis of recent child-training literature. In M Mead & M Wolfenstein (Eds) *Childhood in Contemporary Cultures*. Chicago: The University of Chicago Press. Reprinted in H Jenkins (Ed) (1998) *The Children's Culture Reader* (pp 199–208). New York: NYU Press.

8. See Richards, B (1989) Visions of freedom. *Free Association, 16*, 31–42, for an explanation of the psychological mechanisms behind this.

9. Scheper-Hughes, N & Stein, HF (1987) Child abuse and the unconscious in American popular culture. In N Scheper-Hughes (Ed) *Child Survival* (pp 339–58). New York: D Reidel Publishing.

10. Timimi, S (2005) *Naughty Boys: Anti-social behaviour, ADHD, and the role of culture*. Basingstoke: Palgrave MacMillan; and Timimi, S (2007) *Misunderstanding ADHD: A complete guide for parents to alternatives to drugs*. Milton Keynes: AuthorHouse.

11. See UNICEF (2007) *An Overview of Child Well-Being in Rich Countries*. Florence: UNICEF Innocenti Research Centre; and The Children's Society (2008) *The Good Childhood Inquiry Reveals Mounting Concern over the Commercialisation of Childhood*. Available at <http://www.childrenssociety.org.uk/whats_happening/media_office/latest_news/6486_pr.html>. Accessed 04.03.2008.

12. Stephens, S (1995) Children and the politics of culture in 'Late Capitalism'. In S Stephens (Ed) *Children and the Politics of Culture* (pp 3–50). Princeton, NJ: Princeton University Press.

13. Maitra, B (2006) Culture and the mental health of children. The 'cutting edge' of expertise. In S Timimi & B Maitra (Eds) *Critical Voices in Child and Adolescent Mental Health* (page numbers of chapter pp 48–74). London: Free Association Books.

14. Timimi, S (2005) *Naughty Boys: Anti-social behaviour, ADHD, and the role of culture*. Basingstoke: Palgrave MacMillan.

15. Ang, I (1996) *Living Room Wars*. London: Routledge.

16. Stephens, S (1995) Children and the politics of culture in 'Late Capitalism'. In S Stephens (Ed) *Children and the Politics of Culture*. Princeton, NJ:

Princeton University Press, 1995.

17. Wong, IC, Murray, ML, Camilleri-Novak, D & Stephens, P (2004) Increased prescribing trends of paediatric psychotropic medications. *Archives of Disease in Childhood, 89*, 1131–2.

18. Timimi, S (2005) Effect of globalisation on children's mental health. *British Medical Journal, 331*, 37–9.

19. Fernea, EW (Ed) (1995) *Children in the Muslim Middle East*. Austin, TX: University of Texas Press.

20. Banhatti, R, Dwivedi, K & Maitra, B (2006) Childhood: An Indian perspective. In S Timimi & B Maitra (Eds) *Critical Voices in Child and Adolescent Mental Health*. London: Free Association Books.

Chapter 3

1. Available at <http://www.rcpsych.ac.uk/mentalhealthinformation/mentalhealthandgrowingup/5adhdhyperkineticdisorder.aspx>. Accessed 03.03.2008

2. Or Hyperkinetic disorder as it used to be known in the UK, which traditionally used a different diagnostic (*International Classification of Diseases – ICD*) manual to the USA (which uses *Diagnostic and Statistical Manual – DSM*). Nowadays Hyperkinetic disorder is rarely used as a diagnosis, even in the UK; the preference being for using ADHD.

3. American Psychiatric Association (1994) *Diagnostic and Statistical Manual of Mental Disorders,* (4th ed) *(DSM-IV)*. Washington DC: APA.

4. See Romme, M & Escher, S (Eds) (1993; 2nd ed, 1998). *Accepting Voices*. MIND Publications, London; and Escher, S & Romme, M (1998) Small talk: Voice-hearing in children. *Open Mind,* July/August.

5. You can find detailed arguments and full references in my previous books (written for an academic and professional audience): Timimi, S (2002) *Pathological Child Psychiatry and the Medicalization of Childhood.* London: Routledge-Brunner; Timimi, S (2005) *Naughty Boys: Anti-social behaviour, ADHD and the role of culture.* Basingstoke: Palgrave MacMillan; Timimi, S & Begum, R (Eds) (2006) *Critical Voices in Child and Adolescent Mental Health.* London: Free Association Books; and in Timimi, S (2007) *Misunderstanding ADHD: A complete guide for parents to alternatives to drugs.* Milton Keynes: AuthorHouse, written for parents and carers.

6. For example: Battle, ES & Lacey, B (1972) A context for hyperactivity in children over time. *Child Development, 43*, 757–73.

7. For a summary, see Taylor, E (1994) Syndromes of attention deficit and overactivity. In M Rutter, E Taylor & L Hersov (Eds) *Child and Adolescent*

Psychiatry: Modern approaches (3rd edn) (pp 285–307). Oxford: Blackwell Scientific Publications.

8. Rappley, MD, Gardiner, JC, Jetton, JR & Howang, RT (1995) The use of methylphenidate in Michigan. *Archives of Pediatric and Adolescent Medicine, 149*, 675–9.

9. Pillia, A, Patel, V, Cardozo, P, Goodman, R, Weiss, H, & Andrew, G (2008) Non-traditional lifestyles and prevalence of mental disorders in adolescents in Goa, India. *British Journal of Psychiatry, 192*, 45–51.

10. See <http://www.adhdrelief.com/famous.html>. Accessed 03.03.2008.

11. Castellanos, FX, Lee, PP, Sharp, W et al (2002) Developmental trajectories of brain volume abnormalities in children and adolescents with attention-deficit/hyperactivity disorder. *Journal of the American Medical Association, 288*, 1740–8.

12. For further discussion, see Leo, JL & Cohen, DA (2003) Broken brains or flawed studies? A critical review of ADHD neuroimaging research. *The Journal of Mind and Behavior, 24*, 29–56.

13. See for example: Kitayama, N, Quinn, S & Bremner, JD (2006). Smaller volume of anterior cingulate in abuse-related posttraumatic stress disorder. *Journal of Affective Disorders, 90*, 171–4; and Teicher, MH, Tomoda, A & Andersen, SL (2006) Neurobiological consequences of early stress and childhood maltreatment: Are results from human and animal studies comparable? *Annals of the New York Academy of Sciences, 1071*, 313–23; and Kaufman, J & Carney, D (2001) Effects of early stress on brain structure and function: Implications for understanding the relationship between child maltreatment and depression. *Development and Psychopathology, 13*, 451–71.

14. For further discussion, see Carey, WB & McDevitt, SC (1995) *Coping with Children's Temperament: A guide for professionals.* New York: Basic Books.

15. Barkley, R et al (2002) International consensus statement on ADHD. *Clinical Child and Family Psychology Review, 5*, 89–111.

16. For all the up-to-date research on ADHD genetics see Joseph, J (2006) *The Missing Gene: Psychiatry, heredity, and the fruitless search for genes.* New York: Algora. A summary is also provided in my book, Timimi, S (2007) *Misunderstanding ADHD: A complete guide for parents to alternatives to drugs.* Milton Keynes: AuthorHouse.

17. Available at <http://www.rcpsych.ac.uk/mentalhealthinformation/ mentalhealthandgrowingup/34depressioninchildren.aspx>. Accessed 03.03.2008.

18. American Psychiatric Association (1994) *Diagnostic and Statistical Manual of Mental Disorders* (4th ed) *(DSM-IV).* Washington, DC: APA.

19. Hill, P (1997) Child and adolescent psychiatry. In R Murray, P Hill & P McGuffin (Eds) *The Essentials of Postgraduate Psychiatry* (3rd edn) (pp 97–143). Cambridge: Cambridge University Press.

20. Harrington, R (1994) Affective disorders. In M Rutter, E Taylor & L Hersov (Eds) *Child and Adolescent Psychiatry: Modern approaches* (3rd edn) (pp 330–50). Oxford: Blackwell Scientific Publications.

21. Pickles, A, Rowe, R, Simonoff, E, Foley, D, Rutter, M & Silberg, J (2001) Child psychiatric symptoms and psychosocial impairment: Relationship and prognostic significance. *British Journal of Psychiatry, 179*, 230–53.

22. Harrington, R, Fudge, H, Rutter, M, Bredenkamp, C, Groothues, C & Pridham, J (1993) Child and adult depression: A test of continuities with data from a family study. *British Journal of Psychiatry, 162*, 627–33.

23. Timimi, S (2004) Rethinking childhood depression. *British Medical Journal, 329*, 1394–6.

24. See Timimi, S (2006) Childhood depression? In S Timimi & B Maitra (Eds) *Critical voices in child and adolescent mental health* (pp 200–13). London: Free Association Books, for further discussion about childhood depression.

25. American Psychiatric Association (1994) *Diagnostic and Statistical Manual of Mental Disorders* (4th ed) *(DSM-IV)*. Washington DC: APA.

26. See <http://www.nas.org.uk/nas/jsp/polopoly.jsp?d=10>. Accessed 03.03.2008.

27. Rutter, M, Andersen-Wood, L, Beckett, C et al, and the autistic patterns following severe early global privation. *Journal of Child Psychology and Psychiatry, 40*, 537–49.

28. Lotter, V (1966) Epidemiology of autistic conditions in young children, I. Prevalence. *Social Psychiatry, 1*, 124–37.

29. See <http://www.nas.org.uk/nas/jsp/polopoly.jsp?d=10>. Accessed 03.03.2008

30. Nadesan, M (2005) *Constructing Autism: Unravelling the 'truth' and understanding the social*. London: Routledge.

31. Lotter, V (1966) Epidemiology of autistic conditions in young children, I. Prevalence. *Social Psychiatry, 1*, 124–37.

32. See <http://en.wikipedia.org/wiki/Autism_rights_movement>. Accessed 03.03.2008.

33. LeVine, RA, Dixon, S, LeVine, S, Richman, A, Leiderman, PH, Keefer, CH & Brazelton, TB (1994) *Child Care and Culture: Lessons from Africa.* Cambridge: Cambridge University Press.

Chapter 4

1. See the special issue of the British Medical Journal on May 31st, 2003. *British Medical Journal, 326*, 1155–222.

2. Mintzes, B (2002) Direct to consumer advertising is medicalising normal human experience. *British Medical Journal, 324*, 908–11.

3. Boyd, EA & Bero, LA (2000) Assessing faculty financial relationships with industry. *Journal of the American Medical Association, 284*, 2209–14.

4. Wazana, A (2000) Physicians and the pharmaceutical industry. Is a gift ever just a gift? *Journal of the American Medical Association, 283*, 373–80.

5. Kmietowicz, Z (2005) NHS criticised for lax control over drugs industry. *British Medical Journal, 330*, 805.

6. Quoted from Hearn, K (2004) Here kiddie, kiddie. Available at <http://alternet.org/drugreporter/20594/>. Accessed 03.03.2008.

7. See <http://www.adders.org/news91.htm>. Accessed 03.03.2008.

8. See for example, Schachter, H, Pham, B, King, J, Langford, S & Moher, D (2001) How efficacious and safe is short-acting methylphenidate for the treatment of attention-deficit disorder in children and adolescents? A meta-analysis. *Canadian Medical Association Journal, 165*, 1475–88; and M McDonagh & K Peterson (2005) *Drug class review on pharmacological treatments for ADHD*. Portland OR: Oregon Health and Science University.

9. See <http://health.usnews.com/usnews/health/articles/070221/21.ritalin.htm>. Accessed 03.03.2008.

10. See Joughin, C & Zwi, M (1999) *Focus on the Use of Stimulants in Children with Attention Deficit Hyperactivity Disorder. Primary Evidence-Base Briefing No.1*. London: Royal College of Psychiatrists Research Unit; and Timimi, S (2006) The politics of Attention Deficit Hyperactivity Disorder. In S Timimi & B Maitra (Eds) *Critical Voices in Child and Adolescent Mental Health* (pp 171–99). London: Free Association Books.

11. MTA Co-operative Group (1999) A 14-month randomized clinical trial of treatment strategies for attention deficit/hyperactivity disorder. *Archives of General Psychiatry, 56*, 1073–86.

12. See Boyle, MH & Jadad, AR (1999) Lessons from large trials: The MTA study as a model for evaluating the treatment of childhood psychiatric disorder. *Canadian Journal of Psychiatry, 44*, 991–8; and Breggin, P (2000) The NIMH multimodal study of treatment for attention deficit/hyperactivity disorder: A critical analysis. *International Journal of Risk and Safety in Medicine, 13*, 15–22.

13. MTA Co-operative Group (2004) National Institute of Mental Health Multimodal Treatment Study of ADHD follow-up: 24-month outcomes of treatment strategies for attention-deficit/hyperactivity disorder. *Pediatrics, 113*, 754–61.

14. Jensen, P, Arnold, E, Swanson, J, et al (2007) Three-year follow-up of the NIMH MTA study. *Journal of the American Academy of Child and Adolescent Psychiatry, 46*, 988–1001.

15. Quoted from Hearn, K (2004) Here kiddie, kiddie. Available at <http://alternet.org/drugreporter/20594/>. Accessed 03.03.2008.

16. See for example, Babcock, Q & Byrne, T (2000) Student perceptions of methylphenidate abuse at a public liberal arts college. *Journal of American College Health, 49*, 143–5; and Teter, C et al (2003) Illicit methylphenidate use in an undergraduate student sample: Prevalence and risk factors. *Pharmacotherapy, 23*, 609–17.

17. Volkow, ND, Ding, YS, Fowler, JS et al (1995) Is methylphenidate like cocaine. *Archives of General Psychiatry, 52*, 456–63.

18. For further discussion of the research in this area, see Jackson, G (2005) *Rethinking Psychiatric Drugs*. Bloomington IN: AuthorHouse.

19. Birmaher, B, Ryan, N, Williamson, D, Brent, D & Kaufman, J (1996) Childhood and adolescent depression: A review of the past 10 years. Part II. *Journal of the American Academy of Child and Adolescent Psychiatry, 35*, 1575–1583.

20. Jureidini, J, Doecke, C, Mansfield, P, Haby, M, Menkes, D & Tonkin, A (2004) Efficacy and safety of antidepressants for children and adolescents. *British Medical Journal, 328*, 879–83.

21. Craig, J, Whittington, CJ, Kendall, T, Fonagy, P, Cottrell, D, Cotgrove, A & Boddington, E (2004) Selective serotonin reuptake inhibitors in childhood depression: Systematic review of published versus unpublished data. *Lancet, 363*, 1341–5.

22. *CG28 Depression in children and young people: NICE guideline*. National Institute for Health and Clinical Excellence, 2005.

23. Treatment for Adolescents with Depression Study Team (2004) Fluoxetine, cognitive-behavioral therapy, and their combination for adolescents with depression: Treatment for Adolescents with Depression Study (TADS) randomized controlled trial. *Journal of the American Medical Association, 292*, 807–20.

24. Jureidini, J, Tonkin, A & Mansfield, P (2004) TADS study raises concerns. *British Medical Journal, 329*, 1343–4.

25. Duncan, B, Miller, S, Sparks, J, Jackson, G, Greenberg, R & Kinchin, K (2004) The myth of the magic pill. In B Duncan, S Miller & J Sparks *The Heroic Client* (pp 147–77). San Francisco, CA: Jossey-Bass.

26. See Leo, J (2006) The truth about academic medicine: Children on psychotropic drugs and the illusion of science. In S Timimi & B Maitra (Eds) *Critical Voices in Child and Adolescent Mental Health* (pp 115–35). London: Free Association Books.

27. See for example, Koplewicz, H (1997) *It's Nobody's Fault: New hope and help for difficult children and their parents*. New York: Three Rivers Press.

28. Moncrieff, J (2008) *The Myth of the Chemical Cure*. Basingstoke: Palgrave MacMillan. (2009) *A Straight-Talking Introduction to Psychiatric Drugs*, pp. 31–52. Ross-on-Wye: PCCS Books.

29. New antipsychotic drugs carry risks for children. *USA Today* 5th February 2006. Available at <http://www.usatoday.com/news/health/2006-05-01-atypical-drugs_x.htm>. Accessed 03.03.2008.

30. Morgan, S & Taylor, E (2007) Antipsychotic drugs in children with autism. *British Medical Journal, 334*, 1069–70.

31. McCracken, JT, McGough, J, Shah, B et al (2002) Resperidone in children with autism and serious behavioral problems. *New England Journal of Medicine, 347*, 314–21; and Shea, S, Turgay, A, Carroll, A et al. (2004) Risperidone in the treatment of disruptive behavioral symptoms in children with autistic and other pervasive developmental disorders. *Pediatrics, 114*, e634–41.

32. <http://www.usatoday.com/news/health/2006-05-01-atypical-drugs_x.htm>. Accessed 03.03.2008

33. Michael, KD & Crowley, SL (2002) How effective are treatments for child and adolescent depression? A meta-analytic review. *Clinical Psychology Review, 22*, 247–69; and Duncan, B, Miller, S & Sparks, J (2004) *The Heroic Client*. San Francisco CA: Jossey-Bass.

34. For a recent and thorough review of this evidence see Wampold, BE (2001) *The Great Psychotherapy Debate*. Mahwah, NJ and London: Lawrence Erlbaum Associates.

35. Duncan, B, Miller, S & Sparks, J (2004) *The Heroic Client*. San Francisco, CA: Jossey-Bass.

Subject index

Index

Name index

Index